GMO & CRISPR Gene-Edited Food Checklist

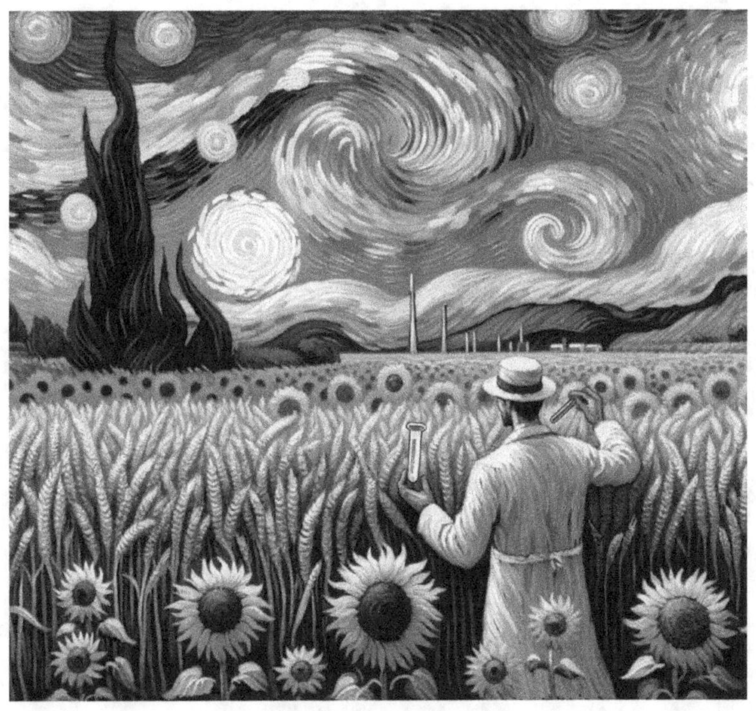

Illustration of a new GMO wheatfield in the style of Van Gogh

"The wheat field has . . . poetry. It is like a memory of something one has once seen. We can only make our pictures speak." **—Vincent Van Gogh**

Alex Jack

GMO & CRISPR Gene-Edited Food Checklist

For further information on special sales, mail-order sales, wholesale distribution, translations, foreign rights, contact the publisher: Planetary Health/Amberwaves Press, PO Box 487, Becket MA 01223 • (413) 623-0012 • shenwa26@yahoo.com

ISBN 9798326708434

10 9 8 7 6 5 4 3 2 1

Contents

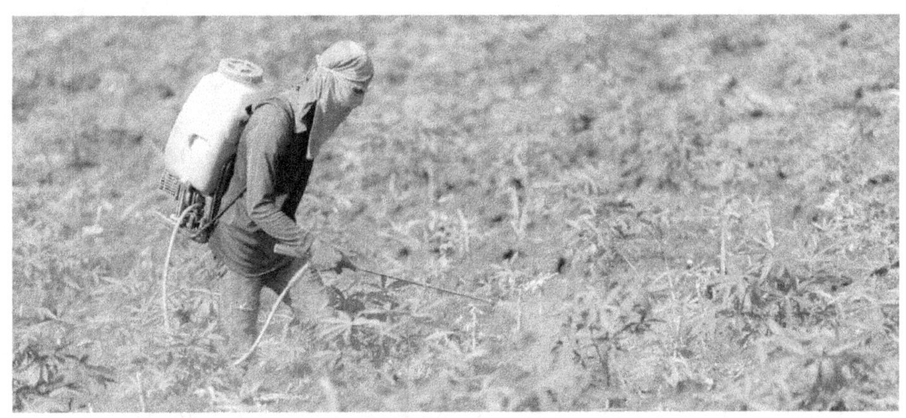

Preface: GMO & Gene-Edited Food

"Genetically modified means an organism in which the genetic material has been changed through gene technology in a way that does not occur naturally by multiplication and/or any natural recombination." – United Nations

Genetically modified organisms (GMOs) have moved almost invisibly into the global food supply over the last generation. In the absence of comprehensive testing, their long-term effects on human health and the environment remain unknown. Short-term studies suggest that they present major risks to human health and the environment.

The American Academy of Environmental Medicine (AAEM) has called on "Physicians to educate their patients, the medical community, and the public to avoid GM (genetically modified) foods when possible and provide educational materials concerning GM foods and health risks." In a policy statement, they called for a moratorium on GM foods, long-term indepen-dent studies, and labeling. AAEM's statement declared, "Several animal studies indicate serious health risks associated with GM food," including infertility, immune problems, accelerated aging, insulin regulation, and changes in major organs and the gastrointestinal system. They concluded, "There is more than a casual association between GM foods and adverse health effects. There is causation."[1] The American Medical Association called for mandatory pre-market safety testing of GMO foods. Hundreds of independent scientific and medical studies around the world have warned of the dangers of GMOs and led to these warnings. (See Section 39 below for a summary of the "The 50 Major Risks of GMOs.")

Like the release of radioactive fallout into the atmosphere from nuclear weapons testing during the Cold War or the widespread use of arsenic, asbestos, and other toxins in household and industrial products, the introduction of foreign genes into natural species of plants and animals or editing within existing genomes constitutes a vast, unregulated intervention and modification of the natural environment. The impact on the food supply, on water, air, and soil quality, and on human culture and civilization has already proved disastrous in some cases and in the long term could be catastrophic.

Like nuclear energy, many environmentalists are beginning to embrace genetic engineering as a green technology. Toyota developed two new GMO flowers to absorb auto emissions. It turned out that producing the Prius hybrid created more carbon dioxide than normal gas vehicles, nullifying the CO_2 savings over the life of the Prius. Toyota disputed these numbers, but in reply to the criticism engineered two species of flowers that absorbed heat and nitrogen oxides (both common pollutants from the Toyota lines) from the atmosphere. Toyota's new flowers were derived from the cherry sage and gardenia, and Toyota reportedly planned to add the altered blooms to the landscaping outside its factory in Toyota City, Japan. Such short-sighted innovations ignore the long-range effect of releasing GMOs into the environment and its effects on other flowers, plants, and wildlife, including bees and other pollinators.

According to polls, more than 90% of the American people are concerned about GMO food and want mandatory labeling. For two decades, the U.S. government steadfastly resisted this measure as unnecessary. It finally bowed to public opinion in 2016 and instituted an opaque system of labeling that only served to further confuse the issue.

Public unease about Big Food, Big Agriculture, and Big Pharma are reflected in popular culture. A key reason the hit film *The Hunger Games* resonated with audiences was because of its depiction of a future world in which GMO wasps, dogs, and other engineered animals and insects enforced conformity and obedience. Another example is the modern Spiderman saga, in which Peter Parker is bitten by a radioactive spider. These entertaining movies are modern myths, reflecting the fear of losing our natural human quality and becoming a hybrid species.

In the absence of accurate and verifiable information, fear, panic, and rumor fill the void. Even knowing what foods and ingredients are genetically altered is a mystery today to most people. In 2000, Planetary Health published its first guidebook on this subject entitled *Imagine a World Without Monarch Butterflies: Awakening to the Hazards of Genetically Altered Foods*. In the foreword to this book, Congressman Dennis J. Kucinich wrote: "The human heart is very powerful, and the human soul is unconquerable. One person who holds fast to his or her ideals and strives for justice in the face of seemingly impossible odds can stir the transformation of social, political, and economic structures. This is why markets will change. This is why genetically engineered products will be labeled. We must always believe in our ability to change things. One person can make a difference."

New Gene-Edited Foods

The global dietary and nutritional landscape was further disrupted in the early 2020s by a new class of genetically engineered foods derived from NGT plants. NGT stands for New Genomic Techniques, a new form of genetic technology that can be used to "edit" genes within plants, animals, humans, and other organisms. It makes use of CRISPR, an acronym for "clustered regularly interspaced palindromic repeats," that uses genetic sequencing to identify and open specific strands of complementary DNA. The first generation of GMOs combined *two species*, splicing genetic material from one and inserting it into another. CRISPR, the second generation, alters, combines, and reformulates genetic material within the same or *one species*.

In both cases, few if any comprehensive safety tests on human health or the environment have been conducted. If GMO labeling is opaque, that for NGT is nonexistent. Governments have barely addressed the complex issues they pose. In the U.S., they must be approved by the FDA, but they are unlabeled, since, unlike GMOs, they do not cross species boundaries.

The potential for harm is alarming. In 2018, Chinese physician He Jiankui altered the DNA of two human embryos leading to the birth of the world's first two gene-edited babies. The procedure was botched, carried out secretly, and the parents of the little girls were misled about the nature of the procedure. The resulting scandal horrified most scientists, leading to an unofficial moratorium on gene-editing humans.

Studies of NGT or CRISPR-altered plants have given scientists reason to doubt the precision and value of the new technology. For example, scientists began to experiment with gene-editing poplar trees, a common ornamental. Usually, the plants take seven to ten years to flower in nature. After "gene scissors" based interventions, they flowered after just four months. Environmentalists pointed out that poplar is a key source of food for beetles, butterflies, bees, and other pollinators. If GMO trees cross, or interbreed, in the wild, the natural poplar population may collapse as the new traits are not adapted to the environment. As ecologists warned, once edited and released into nature, the genes are irreversible and cannot be recalled like a defective product.

In Japan, one of the first CRISPR edited foods, the GABA tomato, was released in 2023. According to the manufacturer, the tomatoes will lower blood pressure, relieve mental stress, and improve sleep quality. The amount of gamma aminobutyric acid (GABA) in the altered tomatoes was reportedly from 4 to 6 times higher than in conventionally bred varieties. GABA is the chief inhibitory neurotransmitter in the mammalian central nervous system and reduces neuronal excitability. It is used in drugs to increase relaxation, reduce anxiety, and prevent convulsions. On the downside, it can cause increased heart rate, muscle weakness, nausea, headache, and amnesia. Clinical research found that GABA supplementation did not reduce stress or enhance sleep quality.[2]

The limitations, errors, and mishaps of gene-editing continued to accumulate. A review of CRISPR studies on human, primate, and mouse cells from Rice University found that the splicing technology caused numerous large unintended on-target genetic damages, including large and small deletions and insertions and chromosomal rearrangements of genetic material. *Base editing* and *prime editing*—two recent CRISPR applications—cause single strand breaks in DNA instead of double-strand breaks and are less prone to DNA repair, also leading to large deletions, insertions, and rearrangements.[3] As British geneticist Michael Antoniou declared, "It has become clear from the accumulating evidence that in terms of unintended outcomes, gene editing appears no better than gene additional gene therapy. In gene addition gene therapy, you have very low frequency insertional mutagenesis with a possible cancer outcome. In this context, gene editing could even be riskier than gene addition."[4]

While genetically editing humans remains temporarily off limits, it is rapidly moving ahead with animals as well as plants. The problem with germline editing is that the unintended consequences are inherited in subsequent generations. In one trial, an attempt to manipulate the genes of cattle to produce only the birth of male calves went terribly awry. The only calf to survive turned out to have seven copies of the targeted gene inserted into its DNA instead of one. Two of these were inserted backwards, and the entire bacterial plasmid DNA construct that carried the male gene was inserted rather than only the desired sequence.[5]

In Israel, researchers gene-edited hens so that they did not produce male offspring. A lethal gene was passed along to male chicks that caused them to die in the egg before they hatch. If the deadly gene escaped into the ordinary chicken population, it could cause havoc, conceivably leading to the collapse of the natural chicken genome. The harmful consequences of this new, untried technology led George Church, a genetics pioneer at Harvard, to call CRISPR "a blunt axe" whose use is "genome vandalism."[6]

Despite these setbacks and failures, the biotech industry continues aggressively to promote CRISPR and other NGT gene-edited foods as precise, safe technologies that did not need to go through biosafety evaluations or be regulated. They have succeeded in Argentina, Brazil, Chile, Colombia, Paraguay,

Honduras, and Guatemala where American agribusiness dominates national politics and the economy. "These new forms of gene manipulation must not be allowed anywhere near our food systems or into the wider environment," stresses Silvia Ribeiro, director of ETC Group in Mexico City.[7]

The U.S. deregulated NGTs in 2018 and Canada in 2023. In early 2024, the European Parliament narrowly voted to deregulate NGT plants that were considered equivalent to conventional plants, while others must comply with current GMO regulation. Several countries, including Germany and Slovakia, Poland, Austria, Belgium, Bulgaria, Luxembourg, Slovenia, Croatia, Romania, and Hungary, opposed the deregulation. The deregulation group included an estimated 94% of NGTs.

The gene-editing process is also known as *synthetic biology* and involves artificially constructing genetic material such as DNA to create new forms of life or to attempt to "reprogram" existing organisms. The U.S. government, including the FDA and USDA, now use the term "bioengineered" in labeling instead of "GMO" or "genetic engineering" to further obscure what's in our food.

GMO & CRISPR Gene-Edited Food Checklist provides the first comprehensive listing of both GMO and CRISPR foods, plants, animals and their products. We hope that this handbook will contribute to clarity on what is safe to eat and what is not.

Over the last year, GMO wheat was commercialized for the first time in Argentina and will soon spread to other countries. Wheat is the staple food for nearly half the globe, and the release of GMO wheat poses an unparalleled threat to the natural food system, human health, and wildlife. (See Chapter 41 for concise information about its release and impact.)

We encourage you to support Amberwaves' ongoing campaigns to preserve rice, wheat, and other foods from genetic engineering, climate change, and mounting environmental threats and to keep America and the planet beautiful.

Alex Jack
Dubnica Nad Vahom, Slovakia
May 17, 2024

1. GMOs by Many Other Names

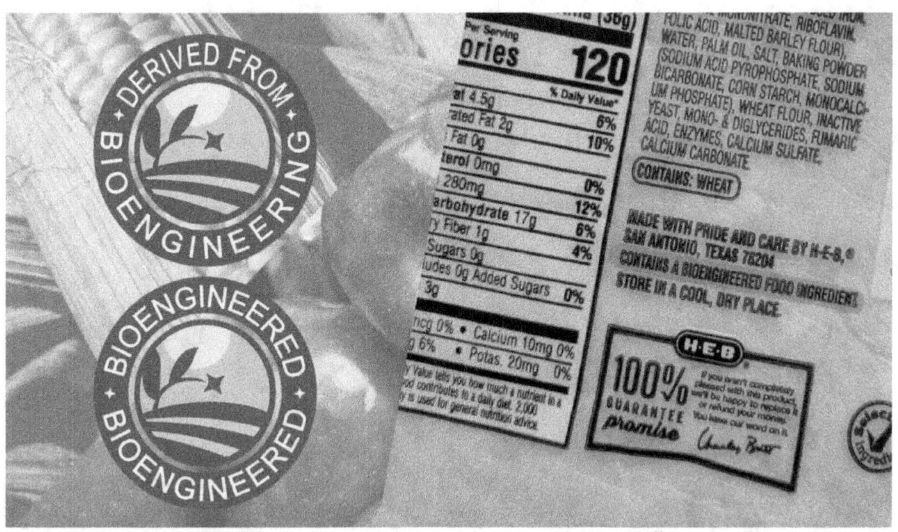

New U.S. labeling law now requires GMO foods or ingredients to be labeled "bioengineered" or include a seal

The United States Department of Agriculture (USDA), Food and Drug Administration (FDA), and Environmental Protection Agency (EPA) have a long history of resisting comprehensive testing and labeling of genetically engineering ingredients.

Certified organic food, by definition, does not generally include GMOs (though there are exceptions, see p. 13). In 2016, Congress passed the National Bioengineered Food Disclosure Standard in response to decades of activism by health, environmental, and medical groups.

The new standard took effect in 2022 and required food makers, importers, and certain retailers to label foods that are genetically engineered or have GMO ingredients. Instead of "GMOs," a term almost universally known, the new labeling law mandated use of the weaker term "bioengineered." Such foods must have information on their packaging using one of three approved methods, including text on the package that states "bioengineered food," the bioengineered food symbol, or a QR code that consumers could click on their smartphone to find the information online. Later that year, following a lawsuit by the Center for Food Safety, a U.S. District Court ruled that the USDA's decision to allow GMO foods to only be labeled with a QR code was unlawful as it hindered consumer access with burdensome digital disclosures.

Many food manufacturers continue to ignore proper labeling or use even more deceptive terms to hide the fact that they are genetically engineered. Virtually none uses the bioengineered label to call attention to their products.

The terms they use to obfuscate their ingredients include:

- Bioactive
- Bioengineered
- Biodesigned
- Biofermented
- Bioidentical
- Precision fermentation
- Precision engineered
- Synbio
- Synthetic biology
- Synthetic ingredients
- Transgenic
- Transgene-free

2. Foods and Ingredients Exempt from Nutritional Labeling

The FDA exempts from all nutritional labeling requirements, including GMO ingredients, for the following foods:

- Dietary Supplements
- Egg cartons (selected)
- Fish
- Food served in bulk containers at a retail establishment. The retail establishment must include the ingredients listing on a card or sign, if not on the bulk container itself
- Foods in small packages that have a total surface area of less than 12 square inches
- Foods served or delivered for immediate consumption
- Foods that are prepared inside a retail establishment and *only* sold in that establishment, e.g., delis, bakeries, or salad bars
- Foods that contain insignificant amounts of all nutrients required to be in a nutrition panel (i.e. coffee beans, tea leaves, spices, flavor extracts, food colors)
- Infant Formula and foods for children up to 4 years of age
- Ingredients that are added to a food for an effect in processing but are present in the finished product at insignificant levels (including many flavorings, enzymes, vitamins, and other additives)
- Packaged single-ingredient meat products that are FDA-regulated (i.e. deer, bison, rabbit, quail, wild turkey, ostrich)
- Raw Fruits
- Some products that are being transported to another facility where they will be processed, packed, or labeled.
- Vegetables

Further, food produced by the following businesses are exempt:

- Businesses that make no more than $500,000 in annual gross sales of all products or that make not more than $50,000 annually in food sales.
- Businesses with fewer than 100 full-time employees and fewer than 100,000 units sold in the U.S.

3. Four Essential Steps to Avoid GMOs & Gene-Edited Foods

The USDA label (left) and the Non-GMO Project label (right) indicate that a food or product is not genetically engineered

1. Buy Organic

All food marketed as organic in the U.S. must be certified by the U.S.D.A. (Department of Agriculture). By definition, "100% organic" foods cannot contain any GMOs. "Organic" food may contain up to 5% conventionally grown ingredients, but also it may not include GMOs. Foods "made with organic ingredients" require only 70% to be organic, but none of the other 30% can contain GMOs. So, these three types of labels on a product ensure that it is non-GMO and safe to eat. In 2016, the National Organic Standards Board voted unanimously to update U.S. organic standards to exclude ingredients derived from the next generation of gene-edited foods (NGTs).

Some companies, such as Eden Foods, the large macrobiotic and natural foods manufacturer in the U.S., have declined to have their foods certified as organic because they feel the U.S. governments standards are too low. Current standards allow a variety of synthetic additives in organic foods that are question-able. Eden has its own in-house laboratory and rigorously tests for GMOs and contracts with farmers to ensure that all its raw materials are GMO-free. Many small farms also grow organi-cally and non-GMO, but are not certified for ethical or financial reasons. They typically market their foods in farmers' markets and CSAs.

Organically grown crops may be contaminated by GMOs in neighboring farms. It is unclear how widespread contamination from pollen, insects, or microorganisms is, as there is no mechanism within the USDA to deal with this problem. State and federal courts are beginning to address this issue and hold biotech farmers responsible for damages.

2. Look for the Non-GMO Project Label or Other GMO-Free Labels

Many companies now label their foods as "GMO-Free," "Non-GMO," or "Made without Genetically Engineered Ingredients." In some cases, only a single ingredient is mentioned, such as a soy or corn derivative. Look for the Non-GMO Project label. This is a voluntary label with a butterfly image that provides consumers with an independent, third-party verified assurance. To date, almost 50,000 natural and conventional foods use this label, and it offers the best and most trusted information on the quality of a product's ingredients.

3. Avoid High-Risk Ingredients

Avoid products containing soy, corn, canola, cottonseed oil, beet root, or sugar unless they are organic. Up to 70% or more of all processed foods including ingredients made from these five products are GMO. See the list of "Invisible Ingredients" on p. 54 for products to avoid as well as the selected list of companies that may use GMOs on p. 51. "Whole grain" and "multigrain bread" in grocery stores and restaurants are often contaminated. Ideally, make your own foods containing any of these items.

4. Purchase Products Listed in This Checklist

A selected list of companies that are GMO- and CRISPR or gene-edited-free is listed on p. 52. Keep this handy when you shop.

4. Countries Producing GMO Foods

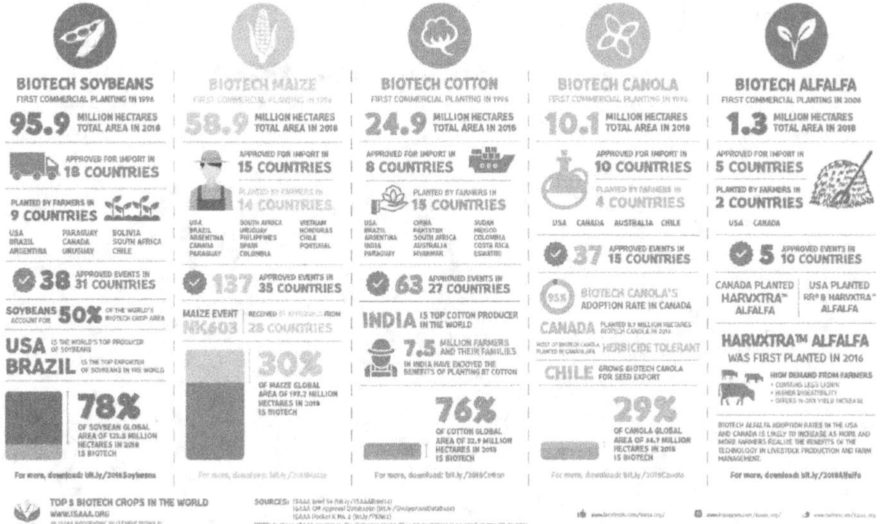

Above: the top 5 GMO crops in the world

- Argentina
- Australia
- Bangladesh
- Bolivia
- Brazil
- Canada
- Chile
- China
- Colombia
- Costa Rica
- Czech Republic
- Ecuador
- Ghana
- Honduras,
- India
- Israel
- Japan
- Kenya
- Malawi
- Mexico
- Myanmar
- New Zealand
- Nigeria
- Pakistan
- Paraguay
- Peru
- Philippines
- Portugal
- South Africa
- Slovakia
- Spain
- Sudan
- eSwatini
- United Kingdom
- United States
- Uruguay
- Vietnam
- Zambia
- Zimbabwe

Restrictions on gene editing in food crops around the world

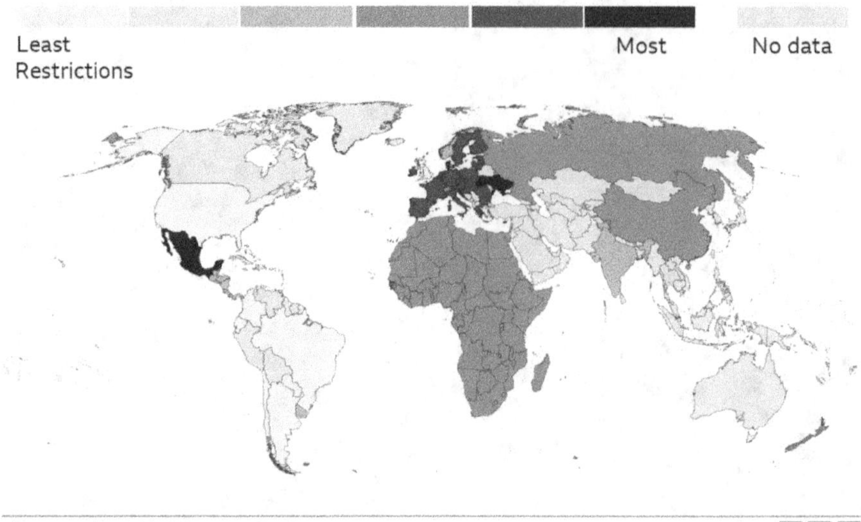

Source: Genetic Literacy Project

B B C

5. Countries with GMO Prohibitions

- **Algeria**: Cultivation banned. Imports banned.
- **Australia**: cultivation prohibited in Tasmania and Kangaroo Island. Imports allowed.
- **Austria**: Cultivation prohibited. Imports allowed.
- **Azerbaijan**: Cultivation banned. Imports allowed.
- **Belize**: Cultivation banned. Imports allowed.
- **Benin**: Cultivation banned.
- **Bhutan**: Cultivation banned. Imports banned.
- **Bosnia and Herzegovina**: Cultivation banned. Imports allowed.
- **Bulgaria**: Cultivation prohibited. Imports allowed.
- **Croatia**: Cultivation prohibited. Imports allowed.
- **Cyprus**: Cultivation prohibited. Imports allowed.

- **Denmark**: Cultivation prohibited. Imports allowed.
- **Ecuador**: Cultivation banned. Imports allowed.
- **France**: Cultivation prohibited. Imports allowed.
- **Germany**: Cultivation prohibited. Imports allowed.
- **Greece**: Cultivation prohibited. Imports allowed.
- **Hungary**: Cultivation prohibited. Imports allowed.
- **India**: Bt cotton allowed, all others prohibited.
- **Italy**: Cultivation prohibited. Imports allowed.
- **Kyrgyzstan**: Cultivation banned. Imports banned.
- **Latvia**: Cultivation prohibited. Imports allowed.
- **Lithuania**: Cultivation prohibited. Imports allowed.
- **Luxembourg**: Cultivation prohibited. Imports allowed.
- **Madagascar**: Cultivation banned. Imports banned.
- **Malta**: Cultivation prohibited. Imports allowed.
- **Moldova**: Cultivation banned. Imports allowed.
- **Netherlands**: Cultivation prohibited. Imports allowed.
- **Northern Ireland, Scotland, Wales** (United Kingdom): Cultivation prohibited. Imports allowed.
- **Norway**: Cultivation prohibited. Imports allowed.
- **Peru**: Cultivation banned (though increasingly ignored). Imports of soy and corn allowed.
- **Poland**: Cultivation prohibited. Imports allowed.
- **Russia**: Cultivation banned. Imports allowed. CRISPR foods are exempt and potato, sugar beet, barley, and wheat are in testing.
- **Saudi Arabia**: Cultivation banned. Imports allowed.
- **Serbia**: Cultivation banned. Imports allowed.
- **Slovakia**: Cultivation banned. Imports allowed.
- **Slovenia**: Cultivation prohibited. Imports allowed.

- **Switzerland**: Cultivation banned. Imports allowed.
- **Turkey**: Cultivation banned. Imports allowed.
- **Ukraine**: Cultivation banned (though law is widely ignored). Imports allowed.
- **Venezuela**: Cultivation banned. Imports banned.
- **Zambia**: Cultivation banned.

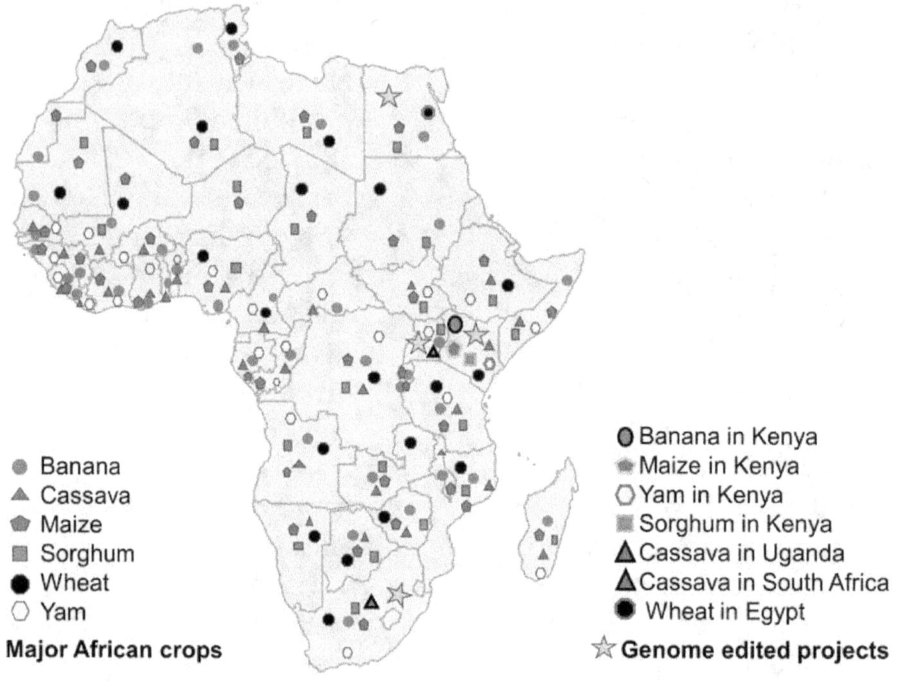

**Map shows where gene-edited trials (CRISPR) are under way in Africa.
Source: Genetic Literacy Project, 2021**

6. CRISPR Gene-Edited Foods

CRISPR and other gene-edited foods entered the marketplace in the late 2010s and early 2020s. Over 600 companies are engaged in synthetic biology developing CRISPR and related gene-edited foods. Since gene-edited foods do not require labelling, they are listed by trait, brand, or developer.

Gene-Edited & Approved

- Apple that is non-browning; marketed as Arctic Apple Fuji, Granny, or Golden varieties (Okanagan Specialty Fruits)
- Avocado - non-browning (GreenVenus)
- Banana – non-browning (Philippines)
- Canola/rapeseed – herbicide-tolerant (Cibus)
- Corn - amylopectin enriched waxy (Corteva Agriscience)
- Corn – waxy (Japan)
- Lettuce - non-browning (GreenVenus)
- Mushroom – white non-browning (Pennsylvania State University)
- Mustard greens - less pungent marketed as Conscious Greens (Pairwise)
- Potato – non-browning (Simplot)
- Pufferfish – fast-growing (Japan)
- Slick-Haired Cattle – with coats that increase resilience to higher temperatures (Acceligen)
- Soybean oil - less fatty (Calyxt)
- Seabream – larger (Japan)
- Surrogate Sires – pork sausages (Washington State University)
- Tomato – GABA enhanced (Japan)
- Wheat – fungal resistant (China)

- Alfalfa – "improved" quality (Calyxt)
- Apple - non-browning Gala, Pink and Honey varieties (Arctic Apple, Okanagan Specialty Fruits)
- Beef (cultured by SciFi and March)
- Camelina – mustard family greens with enhanced omega-3-oil (Yield10 Bioscience)
- Corn - drought-resistant (DuPont)
- Corn - with extra starch (DuPont)
- Cowpea - mechanized harvesting compatible cowpea (Betterseeds)
- Grapes - mildew-resistant wine (Rutgers University)
- Grapes - powdery mildew resistant grapes (VitisGen3)
- Pennycress - high yield (Covercress)
- Potato - non-browning (Calyxt)
- Rice - disease-resistant (Iowa State University)
- Rice – rice blast resistant (Agrotecnio and the University of Lleida, Spain)
- Rice – glutelin reduced (Testbiotech, Japan)
- Rice – rice blast fungus resistant (Testbiotech, Italy)
- Rice - salt-resistant that can be grown in the ocean (Agrisea)
- Soybean - drought- and salt-tolerant (University of Minnesota
- Tomato - high-yield (Cold Spring Harbor Laboratory)
- Tomato - increased antioxidant purple (Norfolk Healthy Produce)
- Tomato - virus-resistant (Nexgen Plants)
- Tomato – miniature for the International Space Station (University of California, Riverside)
- Wheat - high-fiber (Calyxt)
- Wheat - mildew-resistant (Calyxt)

7. Whole Grains

On a global scale, corn or maize is the major genetically modified grain grown and eaten globally. GMO wheat was introduced for the first time in 2023 in Argentina and has been approved by several countries.

All rice is currently non-GMO or non-gene-edited, although many experimental varieties are under development. Golden Rice, the controversial GMO strain designed to combat night blindness, was finally approved for commercialization in the Philippines. However, in 2024 the nation's Supreme Court halted its release pending evidence of its safety following a petition by a coalition of health, environmental, and small rice farmer organizations. All other whole grains are non-GMO.

GMO-Free
- Amaranth
- Barley
- Corn (organic)
- Millet
- Oats
- Rice (except Golden Rice)
- Rye
- Sorghum
- Teff
- Wheat (organic)
- All others

Potentially GMO
- Corn (maize) and corn products
- Rice (only Golden Rice in the Philippines)
- Wheat (Argentinian)

8. Corn and Corn Products

According to the USDA, 92% of the U.S. corn crop, including corn for both animal feed and human consumption, is now engineered. One major type of GM corn contains Bt, a bacteria that releases a toxic protein that is designed to kill the corn borer and other organisms that can damage the crop. However, the plant's pollen can migrate to adjacent milkweed plants and kill the larvae of Monarch butterflies and other beneficial insects. Many processed food products in the supermarket and natural foods store contain corn syrup, cornstarch, corn dextrose, corn oil, corn flour, or other corn product that may be genetically altered. Whole Foods Market (owned by Amazon) was recently targeted by a consumer campaign for carrying bioengineered sweet corn.

GMO-Free
- Organic corn and corn products
- Blue corn
- White corn
- Popcorn
- Baby corn (Chinese style)

Potentially GMO
- Corn dextrose
- Corn flakes
- Corn flour
- Corn masa
- Cornmeal
- Corn oil
- Corn starch
- Corn syrup
- Corn tacos, tortillas, etc.
- Grits
- High fructose corn syrup
- Hominy
- Polenta
- Sweet corn

Processed foods that may contain GMO corn
- Alcohol
- Bread and baked goods
- Breakfast cereal
- Chips
- Condiments
- Cookies & crackers
- Flour
- Fried Foods
- Infant formula
- Mayonnaise & dressings
- Pasta
- Protein powder
- Shortening
- Soups
- Yogurt

---

9. Rice

One variety of GMO rice (LibertyLink) has been approved for sale in the U.S. After several agricultural scandals in the early 2000s involving the contamination of ordinary rice with experimental GMO rice, farmers, the food industry, and many foreign countries objected to its release. Thanks to a national campaign organized by Amberwaves and other health and environmental groups, LibertyLink was never marketed, and there is no GMO rice commercialized in America.

Iran released transgenic rice in 2004, but it was halted two years later, so the world remains GMO-rice free at this time.

Experimental varieties of GMO rice continue to be developed, and some ordinary rice in China has been contaminated by experimental GMO rice that is not legally approved for human consumption.

Non-GMO
• Organic rice
• All other rice in the world except Golden Rice
• Wild rice

GMO
• Golden Rice (a Philippine variety that is currently suspended by the nation's Supreme Court because of health and environmental concerns)
• Rice products from China may have been contaminated with an experimental variety of GM rice that entered the food supply illegally

10. Soybeans and Soy Products

Soybeans, 94% of which are GMO in the USA, are the major biotech beans commercially cultivated. However, they are widely used in ultra-processed foods for the conventional and natural foods marketplace. Soybean oil constitutes 80% of the vegetable oil consumed in America and is used in margarine, salad dressings, mayonnaise, shortening, and other common foods. Many other foods and products contain soy products or derivatives such as lecithin, soy protein, and soy flour.

GMO-Free
- Organic soy and soy products

GMO-Free Tofu, Tempeh, & Other Soy Products Manufacturers
- Franklin's Farms
- House Foods
- Morinaga
- Nasoya
- Nature's Soy
- Pulmone
- Sunrise
- T&T
- Wo Chang

Potentially GMO
- Edamame
- Genistein
- Lecithin
- Miso
- Shoyu
- Soy Flour
- Soy Isoflavones
- Soy Isolates
- Soy Protein
- Soybean Oil
- Soybeans
- Soymilk
- Tamari
- Tempeh
- Tofu
- Veggie burgers

11. Vegetables

With a few exceptions, very few vegetables have been genetically engineered. GMO potatoes were introduced in the U.S. over twenty years ago, but McDonald's rejected them, and the market collapsed. A small volume of GMO potatoes is now grown in Europe. Similarly, a GMO tomato was introduced in the U.S. in the 1990s but failed commercially. An NGT tomato produced in Japan in 2023 is one of the first CRISPR gene-edited foods.

GMO-Free
- Most vegetables with the exception of those noted below
- Organic rapeseed and canola oil products
- Organic squash, crookneck, zucchini and most conventionally grown squashes
- All potatoes, tomatoes, and eggplants grown in the U.S.

GMO
- Papaya (marketed as Rainbow)
- Potato (only in Sweden and Germany)
- Rapeseed (canola grown in the U.S. and Canada)
- Tomato (only in Japan and China)
- Yellow Squash, Crookneck Squash, and Zucchini (small % of the U.S. crop)

12. Fruits and Juices

Papayas from Hawaii, Pinkglow Pineapples, and Arctic Apples are the only fruits currently genetically engineered. However, there is a loophole in the labeling law that exempts GMO food sold or served at food service venues. So whole or pre-sliced fruit or other foods at convenience stores, restaurants, and take out places may be GMO.

Fruit drinks often contain GMO corn syrup, sugar, or HFCS. Dried fruit is commonly sprayed with an oil derived from soybeans that may be GMO. This includes raisins, sultanas, currants, dates, and dried fruit in processed breakfast cereal.

GMO-Free
- Organic fruits and juices
- Organic apples and papaya

GMO
- Arctic Apples
- Papaya from Hawaii (about 80%) and most recently some in Florida
- Pink pineapple

Potentially GMO
- Non-organic dried fruit and juices
- Non-organic sliced fruit

---

13. Seed Oils

About 95% of the rapeseed produced and sold in North America under the name canola oil is GMO. Canola is a popular oil in restaurants and institutional cooking because of its polyunsaturated quality, light texture, and mild taste. It is widely used in processed foods and products. 96% of the cotton crop is GMO and cottonseed oil is widely used in peanut butter, chips, and other processed foods.

GMO-Free
- Organic canola oil
- Organic cottonseed oil
- All other oils

Potentially GMO
- Canola oil
- Cottonseed oil

Processed foods containing GMO oils
- Bread
- Baked Goods
- Cereal
- Chocolate
- Crackers, cookies, chips
- Fried foods
- Infant and toddler formula
- Margarine
- Mayonnaise
- Meat substitutes
- Peanut butter
- Potato chips and others
- Salad dressing
- Veggie burgers

14. Sugar and Sweets

In 2005, the U.S. approved the growing of GMO sugar beets, and 99.9% of the crop is now GMO About half of the sugar consumed in the U.S. comes from sugar beets or more than cane sugar (which is non-GMO) or high fructose corn syrup (which is mostly GMO). GMO sugar was approved in Brazil in 2021 and may be in candy bars and other items.

Honey may also contain GMOs from genetically engineered alfalfa, which was approved by the U.S. government in 2005.

"Sugar" on the label of a product likely indicates a mixture of GMO sugar beets and cane sugar.

The sugar substitute Aspartame is also genetically modified. It is sold under the brand names NutraSweet and Equal and is found in 6000 processed foods, especially diet sodas.

GMO-Free
- Organic sugar and sugar beets
- Organic evaporated cane juice
- Organic Florida crystals
- Organic cola and soft drinks
- Organic honey
- Organic jams, jellies, preserves
- Organic sweets, desserts, and beverages
- Divvies (cookies)

Potentially GMO
- Aspartame (NutraSweet, Equal)
- Dextrin (filler and thickener in sweets, convenience foods, flavoring, vitamins)
- Dextrose (in sweets and energy foods)
- Diet cola
- Fructose (sweetener for diabetics)
- Glucose (used in sweets, baked goods, and soft drinks)
- High fructose corn syrup
- Honey (from rapeseed or alfalfa)
- Jams, jellies, preserves
- Maltodextrin (corn)
- Maltose (used in sugar-free or low-sugar products
- Molasses
- Products made with these ingredients
- Soft drinks
- Stevia
- Sugar
- Sugar beets

15. Milk, Cheese, and Other Dairy Products

About 17% of the cows in the U.S. are in herds given Bovine Growth Hormone (BGH), a GMO growth hormone that increases yields. (It is also known as BST.) In medical studies BGH has been linked with cancer, and it increases mastitis and other diseases in dairy cows. The European Union, Japan, Australia, New Zealand, Argentina, and Canada have banned the use of BGH.

GMO enzymes are also used in an estimated 80 to 90% of cheese produced in the U.S. made with the enzyme rennet. Animal feed commonly consists of GMO corn, soy, and cotton, so many dairy non-organic dairy products include engineered components unless labeled BST or BGH-free.

GMO-Free
- Organic milk & dairy
- Conventional diary
  labeled BGH or BST-free

Potentially GMO
- Butter
- Buttermilk
- Cheese, especially hard
  cheese
- Cream
- Dairy or Soy Cheese made
  with Chymosis or
  Chymax (Rennet)
- Ice Cream
- Milk
- Sour Cream
- Whey
- Yogurt
- Other dairy

Processed foods made with milk or cheese likely to contain GMOs
- Bread
- Cereal
- Candy & cookies
- Margarine
- Pancakes
- Pizza
- Soups

16. Plant-Based Burgers

Many plant-based burgers and other faux meats include GMOs. The Impossible Burger, for example, takes DNA from soybeans and inserts it into a genetically-engineered yeast, which is then fermented to produce heme. Heme gives the food its distinctive red, blood-like coloring and taste.

GMO-Free Burgers, Tofu, etc.
- 365 Brand (Whole Foods)
- Amy's
- Beyond Meat
- Chez Marie
- Beyond Burger
- Boca Burger
- Field Roast
- Follow Your Heart Gardein
- Good Catch (vegan seafood)
- Hilary's Eat Well Lightlife
- Mori-Nu
- Nasoya
- O Organics (Safeway)
- Jackfruit Company Tree of
- Pacific Grains and Foods
- Qrunch Foods
- Small Planet Tofu
- SOL Cuisine
- SoyBoy
- Sunshine Burger
- Sweet Earth Natural Foods
- Wildwood Organic
- White Wave
- Tofurky
- Vitasoy
- WestSoy

GMO Plant-Based Burgers
- Impossible Burger

17. Plant-Based Ice Creams & Milks

Many plant-based ice creams include milk proteins (casein and whey) that are not made from cows but are genetically engineered in high-tech factory farms. Since labeling is not required for proteins, the products are often marketed as animal-free, plant-based, and vegan.

All plant-based milks made from almonds, oats, hemp, and others are non-GMO. An estimated 95% of all soymilks are made from GMO soybeans.

GMO-Free Plant Milks
- Eden Soy

GMO-Free Ice-Cream
- Coolhaus
- Nada Moo
- Divvies

GMO Plant Milks
- 95% of non-organic soymilk

GMO Ice Cream
- Brave Robot Ice Cream
- Graeter's Perfect Indulgence
- Ice Age
- Nick's Vegan
- Perfect Day Vegan Ice Cream
- Smitten Ice Cream

18. Meat, Poultry, Fish, and Other Animal Foods

GMO cattle, sheep, chickens, and seafood are in development, and a few have been approved in the U.S. for human consumption. Except for organic animal foods, almost all meat, diary, poultry, and factory-bred fish in the United States are raised on feed that is genetically altered or contains GMO ingredients. Up to 90% of America's total corn and soybean production goes to feed livestock, and most is GMO. Moreover, 90 to 95% of soymeal, including the outer hulls of the beans, used in human foods are recycled in animal feed. GMO cottonseed oil and cotton byproducts are also added to silage, up to 50% in some cases, and fed to livestock. 94% of the cotton grown in the U.S. is genetically engineered.

GMO-Free
- Wild game
- Wild fish and seafood
- Organically raised animals

Potentially raised on GMO soy or corn ingredients
- Beef, including hamburger, steak, etc.
- Pork, ham, hot dogs
- Lamb
- Chicken, eggs, turkey, and other poultry
- Farm-fed salmon, tilapia, and other fish
- Animals raised on GMO alfalfa

19. Cultured Meat Products

Cultured meat (aka cured meat, vegan meat, etc.) is made from animal cells grown in a lab and does not involve killing an animal. It does not require genetic engineering, though manufacturers may use such techniques to augment its taste, flavor, or other characteristic.

GMO Cultured Meats
- Chicken (Upside Foods)
- Piggy Sooy (Soy-based pork, Moolec Science)
- Motif BeefWorks
- Motif ChickenWorkds
- Motif PorkWorks
- Impossible Burger
- Melt&Marble
- Paleo (Belgium)
- Vegan Mozzarella (New Culture)

20. Beer, Wine, and Alcohol

None of the yeast strains used commercially in fermentation are GM. No GM yeast has been approved in any country. However, GM enzymes may be used in some alcoholic drinks. In the U.S. Anhauser-Busch, makers of Budweiser beer, a rice-based beverage, have helped lead the campaign against GMOs.

GMO-Free
• Budweiser and other Anhauser-Busch beers
• German beers
• Organic beer and wine
• Unibroue beer (Canada)

GMO and Unsafe
• Citizen Original (East Africa)
• Cool Corn (Swiss beer made from Bt maize)
• Kenth (Swedish beer made from Bt maize)

---

21. Flavorings and Colorings

Flavorings and other additives are regulated by the FDA and are labeled as "natural" or "artificial." Artificial may or may not include GMOs.

GMO-Free
- Organic foods

Potentially GMO
- Vanilla
- Citric Acid
- Beta-carotene
- HVP (hydrolyzed vegetable protein)
- Xanthum gum

22. Enzymes

Enzymes are proteins that accelerate biological processes. They are used widely in the food industry to make beer, bread and baked goods, sugar, dairy foods, and other products. Since they are not considered foods, enzymes are not required to be labeled on products. GMO enzymes are unlabeled, and the government does not require that manufacturers notify the FDA. The following GM enzymes are known to have been introduced:

GMO
- Ampha amylase (white sugar, corn syrup, honey)
- Aspartic (cheese)
- Chymosis (cheese)
- Novamyl (bread and baked goods)
- Pullulanase (high fructose corn syrup)

Foods Commonly Made with GMO Enzymes
- Bread and baked goods
- Beer and wine
- Dairy products
- Fruit juices
- Oils
- Sugar

23. GMOs in Restaurant Food

On average, Americans eat out 6 times a week. Up to 70% of all processed foods contain GMO corn, soy, cotton, canola, or sugar beet products or other genetically engineered ingredients.

Many restaurants claim to offer clean and natural food. In a recent test of how glyphosate is prevalent in restaurant food, GMO Free USA, an activist group, tested 44 samples from 38 menu items in a wide range of food options from casual and fast food restaurant chains. Several promoted their food as natural, clean, or superior quality.

The highest levels of glyphosate, a weedkiller used in growing GMO crops and a suspected carcinogen, were detected in "whole grain" or "multigrain" foods. Conventional (non-organic) menu items such as oat-based and wheat-based whole grain breads, bagels, cookies, and pasta were at the highest-risk.

Panera Bread contained the highest level. Panera is one of only two national chains that has pledged to label GMO foods, so this was particularly discouraging. (The other is Chipotle.)

In tests by other organizations over the years, many organic foods have also tested positive for GMOs or glyphosate, showing that certified organic food is widely contaminated in the field or transport. Hence, Panera is probably not deceiving customers. Similarly, Pret a Manger, a popular international chain, promotes its food as "natural" and "free from obscure chemicals," but glyphosate was also found in some of its products in the GMO-Free USA test.

Papa John's Pizza had the highest levels of the chemical among pizzas tested. Samples of food from Whole Foods Bakery, Dunkin' Donuts, Olive Garden, Subway, and McDonalds also tested positive for glyphosate.

GMO Free Restaurants
• Outlets with organic food

Eating Establishments with GMO Ingredients
• Potentially all others

24. Vitamins and Supplements

Several vitamin supplements, especially vitamin C, are commonly made with corn fructose that is genetically altered. Others may be made from corn or soy derivatives.

GMO-Free
- Organic vitamins and supplements

Potentially GMO
- Cysteine (flour treating agent)
- Glutamate (flavor enhancer)

- Natamycin, nisin, and lysozyme (preservatives)
- Vitamin A
- Vitamins B2, B6, B12
- Vitamin C
- Vitamin D and K
- Vitamin E
- Other vitamins and supplements

25. Tobacco

GMO-Free
- Native American Spirit and other organic cigarettes

Potentially GMO
- Commercial cigarettes often include sugar which may be GMO, such as Viceroy, Richland, and Raleigh

26. Cannabis

The difference between hemp and marijuana, which come from the same plant, *cannabis sativa*, is legal, not botanical. A plant with 0.3% or less THC, a psychoactive ingredient, is classified as hemp under U.S. federal law. More than that is considered marijuana.

Cannabidiol (CBD), an active ingredient in cannabis, can be taken internally in the form of inhaling smoke or vapor, oral, and as an aerosol spray into the cheek. CBD oil, an extract from the hemp plant, does not contain THC and has been federally deregulated for public consumption.

GMO hemp has been approved by the FDA for use in growing hemp to further decrease the amount of THC in plants and make them legal for farmers to cultivate.

Many states have legalized marijuana and "medical" marijuana. GMO marijuana is reportedly in development, including new strains that increase THC, but is not yet available commercially.

GMO Cannabis in development
• Hemp (East Fork Cultivars and Phylos Bioscience)
• Hemp - Badger G (University of Wisconsin)
• Marijuana

27. Drugs, Functional Foods, and Other Pharm Foods

The first GMO drug was insulin produced by inserting the human insulin gene into bacteria or yeast cells using recombinant DNA technology.

Functional foods contain some nutrient or compound that boosts nutrition, protects against disease, or has some other other therapeutic use.

Producing drugs in GMO plants is called molecular farming or *biopharming*. There are many potential vaccines under development but not yet released. Some include:

GMO
- Anti dwarfism drugs
- Anti-hemophilia drugs
- Atryn, an anticoagulant made from goat's milk
- Banana, rice, and lettuce for measles
- Corn with anti-contraceptive properties
- Cows spliced with genes to produce human breast milk
- E. Coli with salmonella to produce insulin

- Human breast milk made from cows
- Insulin from bacteria or yeast
- Potato and tobacco for hepatitis B
- Potato for cholera
- Potato for diabetes type 1
- Rice and wheat for cancer
- Tobacco and potato for Norwalk virus
- Tobacco with spinach for rabies
- Tomato for Alzheimer's disease

28. Vaccines

A genetic vaccine or gene-based vaccine contains DNA, RNA, or other nucleic acids that lead to protein biosynthesis of antigens within a cell. DNA vaccines, RNA vaccines, and viral vector vaccines fall under this heading, including most Covid-19 vaccines.

There are other major types of vaccines that are not genetically engineered, including inactivated vaccines (flu shot, polio shot, rabies), live-attenuated vaccines (MMR, smallpox, chickenpox, yellow fever), and toxoid vaccines (diphtheria and tetanus).

Edible vaccines that are spliced right into the food are also on the horizon but not yet available.

GMO Messenger RNA (mRNA) vaccines for Covid
- Pfizer/BioNTech
- Moderna

GMO Viral vector vaccines for Covid
- Oxford/AstraZeneca

GMO Recombinant vaccine for Covid
- Novavax's NVX-CoV2373

GMO Recombinant vaccines
- Cancer
- Ebola
- Hepatitis B
- HIV
- HPV
- HPV (Human papillomavirus)
- Influenza
- Malaria
- Marberg
- Meningococcal disease
- Nipah
- Pneumococcal disease
- Shingles
- Whooping cough
- Others

29. Flowers & Trees

Florigene, part of the Suntory Group, a Japanese company that produces whiskey among other things, brought out the world's first GMO flowers, two varieties of carnation dubbed "Moondust" and "Moonshadow." They have also developed a blue rose that went on sale in Japan. About 50 GMO flowers are in development, the most commonly available are cut blue roses, carnations, lotus, and petunias.

GMO Flowers
- Blue flowers (Moon series carnations or roses)
- Blue rose (Japan and pending in the U.S.)
- Carnation (EU)
- Cherry sage and gardenia (Japan)
- Firefly Petunia
- Lotus flowers – deeper yellow or orange

GMO Trees
- Eucalyptus - Brazil (for papermaking, construction, etc.)
- Poplar – (Living Carbon, U.S., China)

GMO in development
- Algae (Exxon-Mobil, to replace petroleum)
- Bluegrass and other grasses (for hay, ornamental use, golf courses, etc.)
- Chestnut trees
- Orange trees
- Papaya trees
- Pine – loblolly (ArborGen)
- Plum trees
- Rubber trees (India)

30. Animals

Several genetically engineered animals have been introduced as food. Many others are used in research to make drugs, reduce climate change, or serve for general evolutionary research.

GMO Animal-Quality Food
- AquaAdvantage salmon
- GalSafe Pigs (developed by Revivicor for people with meat allergies

GMO animals released into the environment
- Enviro Pig (excretes less phosphorus and reduces dead zones, approved in Canada)
- Mosquitoes that are malaria-, dengue-, or Zika resistant in the Florida Keys and Brazil

GMO Pets
- GloFish

GMO lab animals for drugs or scientific research
- Axolotls, frogs, salamanders, and other amphibians (as pollution sensors and research into tissue regeneration and immunology)
- GalSafe Pigs (organs and tissues for human transplants)
- Green fluorescent cats (for HIV/AIDS research)
- Chickens (mini dinosaur-like phenotypes for evolutionary studies)
- Fruit flies (genetics and inheritance studies)
- Mice (cancer research)
- Marmosets (Parkinson's, ALS, and Hunting's research)
- Rats
- Sea anemone
- Sheep
- Wooly mammoth (extinct genes crossed with the genome of an African elephant for the purpose of rewilding in Siberia and saving the permafrost from climate change; not yet produced)
- Worms (flat, bristle, and others for regeneration studies)

31. Cotton

Ninety-six percent of the cotton grown in the U.S. and 13.5% of cotton grown worldwide is GMO. Besides the U.S., main producers of genetically engineered cotton are China, India, and Pakistan. In 2015, the International Agency for Research on Cancer classified glyphosate, the weedkiller used in growing GMO crops, as a probable human carcinogen.

Only 1% of the world's cotton is organically grown and thus certified as non-GMO. In purchasing fabric, clothing, or other products made from cotton, it is ideal to source organic cotton or conventionally grown cotton products labelled GMO-free. Information on thousands of organic cotton products worldwide is available through the Global Organic Textile Standards public database and the Organic Content Standard certified suppliers list at www.textileexchange.org.

India supplies nearly 50% of the world's organic cotton, followed by China 12.3%,* Kyrgyzstan, 11.8%, Turkey 9.7%, Tanzania 4.5%, Tajikistan 4.2%, and U.S. 2.8%.

Besides clothing, cotton is used in many products, including baby apparel, sheets, pillowcases, towels, footwear, toys, paper, packaging, filling, stuffing, yarn, swabs, cotton balls, tampons, and other medical supplies.

Organic and GMO-Free (selected companies)

- Amour Vest
- Armedangels
- Beaumont Organics
- Bibico
- Boll & Branch
- Brook There
- Christy Dawn
- Continental Cloth
- Cotonea
- Coyuchi
- Dedicated Sweden
- Dibella
- Eileen Fisher
- Fair Indigo
- For Days
- Harvest & Mill
- Industries of All Nations
- Knowledge Cotton Apparel
- Komodo
- Kotn
- Kowton
- Mata Trades
- MATE the Label
- New Nomads
- Nudie Jeans

- Organic Basics
- PACT
- Patagonia
- People Tree
- Tentree
- Thought
- Toad&Co
- Tomboy X
- Veja
- Yes Friends

Potentially GMO Cotton
- China
- India
- Pakistan
- United States

** Warning about Chinese Organic Cotton*

98.5% of the organic cotton grown in China is produced in the Xinjiang region. More than a million native Uyghurs have been removed to "reeducation" camps since 2014 and used as forced labor in the cotton fields and industrial factories. Hundreds of thousands of women have been forcibly sterilized to bring the population down and Islamic religious practices virtually prohibited. The United Nations has found evidence of "crimes against humanity" in Xinjiang, and the U.S. and many other countries have described the systematic eradication of the Uyghur people and culture as genocide.

In purchasing organic cotton products, check the label for the country of origin as many organic products in the U.S., Europe, and other countries may be sourced from China.

32. Body Care, Skin Care & Other Cosmetics

GMO ingredients from corn, soy, canola, and cottonseed oil can be processed into soaps, moisturizers, and other cosmetics. Other botanicals can include GMO yeast, algae, or citric acid.

GMO-Free
- Organic soaps, fragrances, and other cosmetics
- Dr. Bonner's
- Dr. Sheffield's
- Kiss My Face
- Ilia
- Well People

- RMS Beauty
- Merit Beauty
- Jones Road
- 100% Pure
- Alima Pure
- Saie
- Cheekbone Beauty
- Many others

Potentially GMO Body & Skin Care Products
- Bakuchiol
- Butylene glycol
- Cannabioids/CBD/CBG
- Collagen
- Elastin
- Fragrances
- Humetants
- Karatin
- Palm Oil
- ReserveratrolSpider Silk
- Squalone/hemisqualone
- Surfactants
- Vitamins

- Amber
- Ambergris
- Oud/agarwood
- Citrus, orange, grapefruit
- Patchouli
- Vanilla
- Mint

GMO Ingredients in Cosmetics
- AminoSurf-E surfactant (Modular Genetics)
- B-silk (Bolt Threads)
- Brontide butylene glycol (Geno)
- Brontide butylene glycol (Genomatica)
- Collume collagen (Geitor)

Potentially GMO Botanicals
- Sandalwood
- Rose

- Coviance collagen (Geitor)
- ElastaPure elastin (Geitor)
- Hebelys anti-aging extract (Deinove/Greentech)
- Heml5 (Amyis)
- HumaColl21 collagen (Geitor)
- K18Peptide (K18 Hair)
- Luminity neurosporne carotenoid (Delnove)
- Neossane squalene/hemisqualane (Amyris)
- Nootkatone by Evolva (Evolva)
- NovaColl collagen (Cambrium)
- NuColl Pro collagen (Geitor)
- Palmless torula oil (C16 Biosciences)
- Phyt-n-Resist phytoene antioxidant (Deinove)
- Valencene by Evolva (Evolva)
- Veri-te Resveratrol (Evolva)
- Yoil palm oil (Xylome)
- Zemea propanediol (DuPont/Tate & Lyle)

Brands, Developers, and Consortiums Using GMOs
- 4U by Tia Haircare
- AmorePacific
- Aprinnova
- Beebe Lab
- Blossance
- Costa Brazil
- Haeckels the Rewild Body Block Soap
- JLO Beauty
- JVN Hair
- K18Hair L'Oreal
- Nutrinovate Reserol Beauty
- Pipette
- Rose Inc
- Save the F#$%ing Rainforest Body Oil
- Shisido
- The Ordinary
- Vegamour
- Yoil-Cream

33. Seeds

Organic, open-pollinated, or heirloom seeds are non-GMO and are widely available from many large seed companies as well as small speciality suppliers.

The seeds span varieties of grains, vegetables, fruits and berries, seeds, nuts, and other foods as well as high grains, native grasses, cover crops, pasture and lawn seeds, medicinal seeds, culinary herbs and flowers, and wildflowers.

Unless otherwise indicated, the following selected companies are base in the United States:

Organic, Heirloom, or Non-GMO

- Annie's Heirloom
- Baker Creek Heirloom Seeds
- Bejo (Brazil)
- Burpee
- Clear Creek
- DeBolster (Netherlands)
- Eden Brothers
- Fedco Seeds
- Gurney's
- Harris
- High-Mowing
- Johnny's Selected Seeds
- Kisan Agro (India)
- Living Seed Company
- Living Seeds Heirloom Seeds (South Africa)
- McKenzie
- Organic Seeds Australia
- Organicseeds.eu (Europe)
- Peaceful Valley
- Renee's Garden Seeds
- Sahaja Seeds (India)
- Sativa (Germany)
- Seed Savers Exchange
- Seedea (Poland)
- Seeds 'n Such
- Seeds for Africa
- Sementes Vivas (Portugal)
- Southern Exposure
- Sow Diverse (Ireland)
- Sustainable Seed Company
- Territorial Seeds
- The Seedstead (Africa)
- True Leaf

34. Fuel, Ink & Other Non-Food Products

We absorb more than 60% of what our skin comes in contact with, and soy and corn proteins can leave toxic residue on skin, hands, face, etc. Beside cotton and hemp, other products that may contain GMOs include:

Potentially GMO
- Biodegradable plastics (e.g. Biopol from the U.K.)
- Cotton products
- Hand sanitizer
- Hemp products
- Soy ink: used by many natural/eco brands to dye clothing, books, product packaging, print magazines and newspapers and is highly absorbable through the skin
- Spider silk (made from goats which is stronger than steel) used in bullet-proof armor, violin strings, medical bandages, optical fiber cables, and extravagant clothing

- Gasoline: Ethanol 10 and 15 used in ordinary unleaded gasoline contain from 10 to 15% corn ethanol, most of which is GMO
- Vegetable fuel, known as green grease and alternative fuel, is typically recycled from GMO soy and canola oil from restaurants and used as a gasoline or home heating oil substitute

35. Selected GMO-Free Companies and Product Lines

- 365 Brand (Whole Foods)
- After the Fall
- Alta Dena Organics
- Amy's Kitchen
- Anhauser Busch (Budweiser beer)
- Annie's Natural
- Arrowhead Mills
- Baby's Only
- Barbara's (organic line)
- Bearitos/Little Bear
- Ben & Jerry's Ice Cream
- Beyond Meat
- Bob's Red Mill
- Bridge
- Cascadian Farms
- Cliff Bar
- Earth Balance
- Earth's Best
- Eden Foods
- Emerald Cove
- Emperor's Kitchen
- EnviroKids
- Erewhon
- Fantastic Foods
- Gardein
- Garden of Eatin'
- Gerber
- Health Valley (organic line)
- Horizon Organic
- Imagine Foods/Soy Dream
- Imagine Natural
- Kirin Beer
- Knudsen
- Light Life
- Lotus Foods
- Luna Bar
- Lundberg Farms
- Miso Master
- Mitoku
- Moringa
- Muso
- Namaste Foods
- Nasoya
- Natural/Hain
- Nature's Path
- Newman's Own Organics (except salad dressing)
- Odwalla
- Organic Baby
- Pacific Soy
- Rhapsody Foods
- Sapporo Beer
- Seeds of Change
- Silk
- Soy Delicious
- Spectrum Oils
- Stonyfield Farm
- Sun Soy
- Sunshine Burger
- Sweet Cloud
- Tofurky
- Trader Joe's
- Vitasoy
- Walnut Acres
- Westbrae
- White Wave
- Wildwood

36. Selected Companies Using GMOs

- Aunt Jemima (pancakes)
- Balance Bar
- Beech-Nut (baby foods)
- Betty Crocker (meals)
- Blue Sky Natural Beverage
- Boca (meat substitutes, unless organic)
- Campbell's (soups)
- Campbell's (soups)
- Coca-Cola (Fruitopia, Minute Maid, Hi-C, NESTEA)
- Crisco (shortening)
- Duncan Hines (baked goods)
- Enfamil (baby foods)
- FritoLay (chips)
- Gardenburger
- Gerbers
- Green Giant (harvest burger)
- Hawaiian Punch
- Healthy Choice (soups, sauces, canned)
- Heinz (condiments)
- Hellman's (condiments)
- Hershey's
- Isomil and ProSobee (soy formula)
- Kellogg's (corn flakes)
- Kraft (macaroni and cheese)
- Kraft (salad dressings)
- Land O'Lakes (butter, cheese, dairy)
- Lipton (meal packets)
- Lumen Foods (vegetable jerkies)
- Morningstar Farms (meat substitutes, unless organic)
- Nabicso (sundry)
- Nabisco Bars
- Nature Valley (snack and granola bars)
- Near East
- Nestle (baby foods)
- Ocean Spray
- Pasta Roni and Rice-A-Roni (meals)
- Pepperidge Farm
- Pepsi (Tropicana, Frappucchino, Gatorade, Dole)
- Peter Pan (spreads)
- Pillsbury (baked goods)
- PowerBar
- Progresso (soups)
- Quaker Granola Bars
- Quaker Oats (snacks)
- Similiac/Isomil (baby foods)
- Skippy (spreads)
- Smucker's (except for Simply 100% Fruit)
- Soylent (protein power)
- Stouffer's (frozen meals)

37. Invisible GMO Ingredients

Ultra-processed foods frequently have hidden GMO ingredients that are unlabeled, including the following:

Potentially GMO

- Ascorbic acid (vitamin C)
- Aspartame
- Baking powder
- Canola oil
- Caramel color
- Cellulose
- Citric acid
- Colbalamin (vitamin B12)
- Colorose
- Condensed milk
- Confectioners sugar
- Corn flur
- Corn masa
- Cornmeal
- Corn oil
- Corn sugar
- Corn syrup
- Cornstarch
- Cottonseed oil
- Cyclodextrin
- Cystein
- Dextrin
- Dextrose
- Diacetyl
- Diglyceride
- Erythritol
- Equal
- Food starch
- Fructose
- Glucose
- Glutamate
- Glutamic acid
- Glyceride
- Glycerin
- Glycerol
- Glycerol monooleate
- Glycine
- Hemicellulose
- High fructose corn syrup
- Hydrogenated starch
- Hydrolyzed vegetable protein
- Inositol
- Inverse syrup
- Inversol
- Invert sugar
- Isoflavones
- Lactic acid
- Lecithin
- Leucine
- Malitol
- Malt
- Malt syrup
- Malt extract
- Maltodextrine
- Maltose
- Mannitol
- Methycellulose
- Milk powder
- Milo starch
- Modified food starch
- Modified starch

- Mono and diglycerides
- Monosodium glutamate (MSG)
- NutraSweet
- Oleic acid
- Phenylalanine
- Phytic acid
- Protein isolate
- Shoyu
- Sorbitol
- Sly flour
- Sly isolates
- Soy lecithin
- Soymilk
- Soy oil
- Soy protein
- Soy protein isolate
- Soy sauce
- Starch
- Stearic acid
- Sugar
- Tamari
- Tempeh
- Teriyaki marinades
- Textured vegetable protein
- Threonine
- Tocopherols (vitamin E)
- Tofu
- Trehalose
- Trigylceride
- Vegetable fat
- Vegetable oil
- Vitamin B12
- Vitamin C
- Vitamin E
- Whey
- Whey powder
- Xanthan gum

38. The Top 13 Riskiest Foods for Vegans, Macros, and Vegetarians

Most of these risks are faced when eating out in restaurants or purchasing ready-to-eat foods. [7]

1. Veggie burgers, soy burgers, and other vegan items that may include GMO soy, corn, or canola oil. The Impossible Burger is GMO and made from altered blood-like "heme" that gives it "meatiness."
2. "Cultivated," "cultured meat," and "alt-meat"products grown from animal cells in a bioreactor. Though it does not involve killing animals, the lab-grown meat is made from animal cells and is not plant-based. GMO enzymes may or may not have been used because the regulations are inconsistent and there are many exemptions. Manufacturers are not always transparent.
3. Non-organic breads and baked books in food stores and restaurants labeled as "whole grain" or "multigrain"
4. Fried foods that may be made with GMO soy, corn, canola, or cottonseed oil.
5. Vegan mayonnaise with GMO canola oil, peanut butter and other nut and seed butters containing GMO cottonseed oil, and other plant-based foods with GMO soyoil.
6. Commercial or restaurant whole, multigrain, or enriched breads and baked goods that may contain GMO enzymes.
7. Juices, energy drinks, and other beverages made with GMO enzymes.
8. Tofu, tempeh, miso, shoyu, and other soy products made with GMO soy.
9. Dairy (including BGH-free dairy) and other animal products raised on GMO alfalfa or GMO animal feed. Synbio non-animal dairy is made from the blood sample of a cow.
10. Corn, potato, and other chips made with GMO oils.

11. Sweets, desserts, energy bars, and other processed foods containing GMO sugar beets, high fructose corn syrup, fructose, or other derivative. Note: "sugar" on the label usually signifies a combination of GMO sugar beets and non-GMO or GMO cane sugar.
12. Farm-fed salmon, trout, and other fish produced with GMO soy, corn, or cottonseed oil.
13. CRISPR gene-edited foods that are unlabeled and will soon start showing up in stores, restaurants, and other outlets.

39. The 50 Major Risks of GMO & Gene-Edited Foods

This list summarizes the major risks of GMO & Gene-Edited Foods to human health and the environment. Citations from scientific and medical journals for many of these hazards are available in other Planetary Health/Amberwaves publications or online. Documentation is also available from many other sources. Please see Resources for further information.

I. Health hazards
1. Increased allergic reactions and lung problems
2. Increased toxicity and stress on the liver
3. Higher risk of herpes
4. Introduction of foreign proteins in the body
5. Altered or reduced nutrition
6. Damage to stomach, intestines, and blood
7. Impairment of the immune function
8. Increased risk of cancer
9. Increased risk of heart disease
10. Increased risk of diabetes
11. Death and disability
12. Delayed sexuality and reproductive development
13. Increased risk of infertility
14. Increased risk of birth defects and developmental disorders
15. Emergence of antibiotic-resistant bacteria
16. Emergence of new viral diseases

II. Environmental hazards
17. Decline of butterflies and other insects
18. Decline of birds and other wildlife
19. Decline of fish and rise of superfish
20. Increased disease and suffering among animals
21. Contamination of organic crops
22. Contamination of conventional crops
23. Contamination of wild plants
24. Deformed and stunted crops
25. Decline of soil fertility

26. Spread of new viruses
27. Blight, epidemic, and hunger
28. Emergence of of new disease-resistant insects
29. Increased pesticide burden
30. Mutagenesis and inheritance of recessive genes
31. Bioinvasion and irreversible environmental effects

III. Social and cultural hazards
32. Denial of freedom of choice
33. Threat to freedom of speech and other civil liberties
34. Reduced crop yields and economic decline
35. Risky investments and reduced earnings
36. Increased insurance risks
37. Increased world hunger and poverty
38. Patenting of seeds and new life forms
39. Treatment of people as intellectual property
40. Monopoly control and the concentration of wealth
41. Spread of reductionist science and genetic determinism
42. Increased tolerance of ethnic cleansing
43. Increased aggression and violence, especially among Children and adolescents
44. Violent orientation and behavior, including increased hostility toward women, the feminine, and nature
45. Abuse and alteration of language
46. Development of biological weapons and increased risk of bioterrorism and biowarfare

IV. Ethical, religious, and spiritual hazards
47. Playing God and regarding humans as creators of life
48. Violation of traditional dietary codes such as kosher, halal, etc.
49. Danger of genetic apocalypse
50. Violation of natural order

40. Violence, GMOs and UPFs

Consuming GMO foods may be linked to the wave of violence that swept through society, especially the public schools, since the late 1990s. Pesticides, for example, were linked by researchers with a variety of symptoms, including irritability, aggression, and violence.

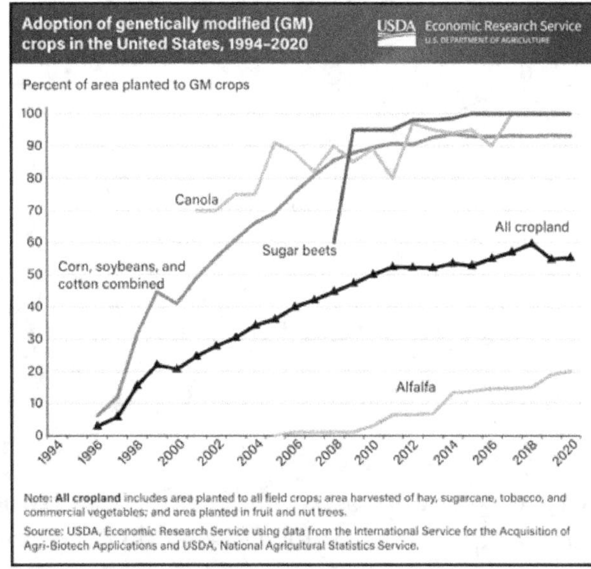

Because of their smaller body mass, children are especially vulnerable to their effects. "A rapidly expanding body of research shows that heavy metals such as lead and pesticides decrease mental ability and increase aggressiveness," Robert Hatherill, a researcher at the University of California, Santa Barbara, wrote in an editorial in the *Chicago Tribune*.[8]

Since about two-thirds of the processed foods and beverages in the school cafeteria contain Bt, a built-in pesticide, or traces of glyphosate, a toxic weedkiller, used in planting genetically engineered crops. GMO foods may be an unrecognized factor in this epidemic of violence. Males are more susceptible than females to pesticides and other estrogen-disrupters. Children, in particular, are exposed to GMO sweeteners and enzymes in breakfast cereals, soft drinks and beverages, juices, cookies, and candy bars. Products containing GMOs included Frosted Flakes, Cap'n Crunch, Count Chocula, Coke, Pepsi, 7-Up, Mountain Dew, Kool Aid, Gatorade, Hawaiian Punch, Oreo Cookies, Fig Newtons, Mounds, Almond Joy, Snickers, Milky Way, and many other well-known brands. Another unrecognized source of genetically engineered pesticides is vitamin C pills. Nearly all the ascorbic acid on the market is made from GMO corn.[9]

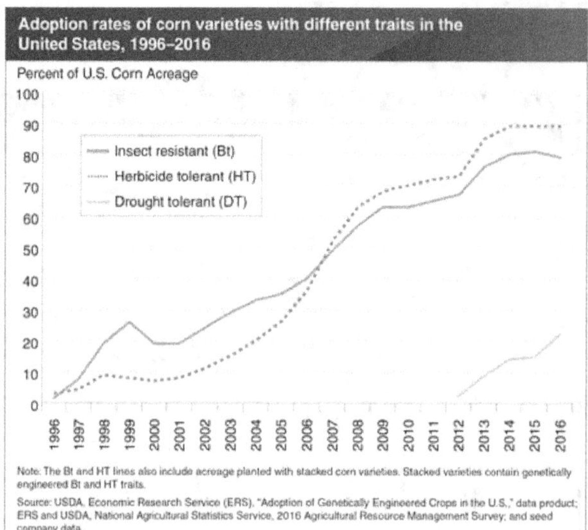

Everyday tens of millions of children and adults pop vitamin C tablets to safeguard their health, yet they may be doing just the opposite.

The Gene Gun

Apart from the pesticide-violence link, teachers, parents, and holistic health practitioners expressed concerned that GMO foods could be a root cause of crimes involving guns, rape, and sexual violence. Contrary to its name and industry persona, genetic engineering is very crude and imprecise. In fact, as the biotech era began, scientists discovered that the hardest part of the engineering process was to get the host organism to accept foreign genes because it was so unnatural. Syringes, chemical solutions, and sophisticated lab techniques used to insert DNA from one organism into another routinely failed.

Since nature was so uncooperative, biotech researchers finally resorted to brute force. Hence the invention of the *gene gun* and the science of *biolistics*. Scientists at Stanford University and the University of California at Davis ultimately achieved the transfer of gene tic material from one organism into another by placing the desired gene in a solution and muzzle-loading it into a pistol shooting modified .22 or .45 caliber bullets. Coated with the DNA to be inserted, these "microbullets" were then fired into a screen covering targeted plant cells and tissue in a petri dish, penetrating the cellulose and dispersing the DNA into the cells.

From the traditional and holistic view of "you are what you eat," we absorb the energy and vibration of the foods we take in, as well as the nutrients and other material components.

60

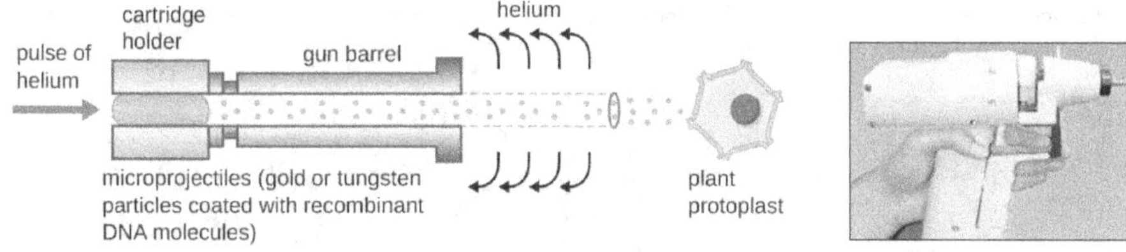

Studies have shown, for example, that plants exposed to Mozart and other classical music grow better than those exposed to rock music and other heavier sounds.[10] The fact that many GMO crops were literally born in the muzzle of a gun, rather than in the peaceful bosom of the earth, should give us pause. It is disturbing to think what energetic effect consuming foods originating from gun-fired DNA will have on human cells and tissues, organs and functions, and minds and consciousnesses. "These foreign genes that could not possibly combine in nature are shot in with a gun—violently," observed Nina Moliver, a Boston nutritionist and women's health practitioner. "It is an act of violence. It supersedes the natural process of sexual repro-duction, so it's anti-sexual in its nature."[11]

Whether increased rape, sexual violence, and prejudice against women and the feminine (e.g., Mother Earth, nature, the intuitive) are on the increase because of the GMOs in our pizza and milkshakes remains to be seen. However, other deficiencies linked with GMO may be contributing to mental and emotional instability in sexual and other matters. According to Monsanto's own research, Roundup Ready lecithin (made from GMO soy) contains 29% less choline than ordinary lecithin.[12] Choline is a vitamin that enhances cognition and other brain functions. Choline-deficient males (or females) are apt to make poor choices and engage in impaired decision making in the home and workplace.

In recent years, biotechnology has become more sophisticated and makes use of viruses and bacteria to insert the genetic material from one species into another. But the gene gun is still used and is often the technology of choice for new gene-editing processes that rearrange the DNA within a single species. An article on "CRISPR'ing Wheat with a Gene Gun" in

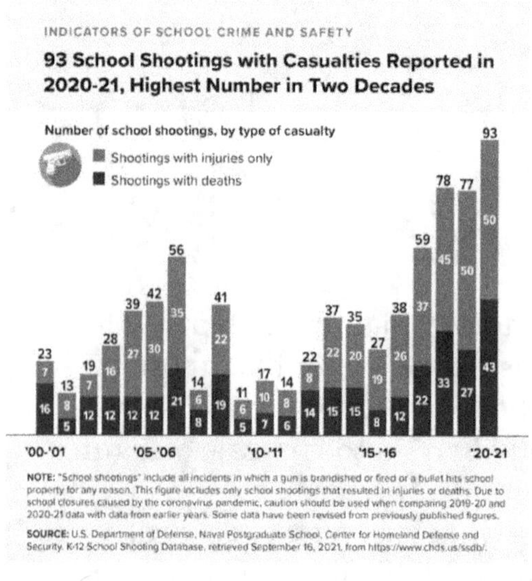

2023 described how scientists "bombarded" wheat embryos with 20 µl of 0.6-micron gold particles. The particles were then "pelleted and resuspended in 20 µl of water. The particles were air-dried onto macro-carrier discs and subsequently used for particle bombardment."

Since the Columbine massacre, there have been more than 400 school shootings in the U.S. exposing 370,000 students to deadly violence. They comprise nearly 60% of all active shooter incidents since 1999. The first wave of shootings coincided with the introduction of GMO foods in the mid-1990s, including items made with ingredients from corn, soy, canola, and cotton. A second wave followed, and between 2010 and 2020, school shootings soared another 1900%.[13] There's been an on-campus shooting "pretty much every single school day" this fall, the founder of the K-12 School Shooting Database said.[14]

This second spike may be linked to the time it takes for GMOs and related toxins to accumulate in the body. The rise in ultra-processed food (UPF) consumption may be another unacknowledged factor. UPFs also soared since 2000 to make up from about 50% of the modern diet to 70 to 80%. A recent study in the *BMJ* (British Medical Journal) concluded: "Greater exposure to ultra-processed food was associated with a higher risk of adverse health outcomes, especially cardiometabolic, common mental disorder, and mortality outcomes."[15] These included mortality from all causes as well as higher risk for type 2 diabetes, heart disease, cancer, respiratory problems, digestive problems, adverse sleep, anxiety, and mental health outcomes. UPFs, which are typically made by reconstituting oil, fat, salt, and protein, along with flavorings, emulsifiers, and other additives, almost always include GMO ingredients among many other harmful substances. These may have driven not only individual acts of violence but also the general polarity in society higher.

It would be premature to directly link the massacre at Columbine High School or the bombing of the World Trade Center by young male terrorists with eating too many GMO-laced burgers, chips, and soft drinks and other ultra-processed foods. But the impact of genetic engineering and food processing on the national and global psyche may be greater than suspected and warrants urgent study.

41. World's First GMO Wheat

This article by Alex Jack originally appeared in Amberwaves, *Summer 2024.*

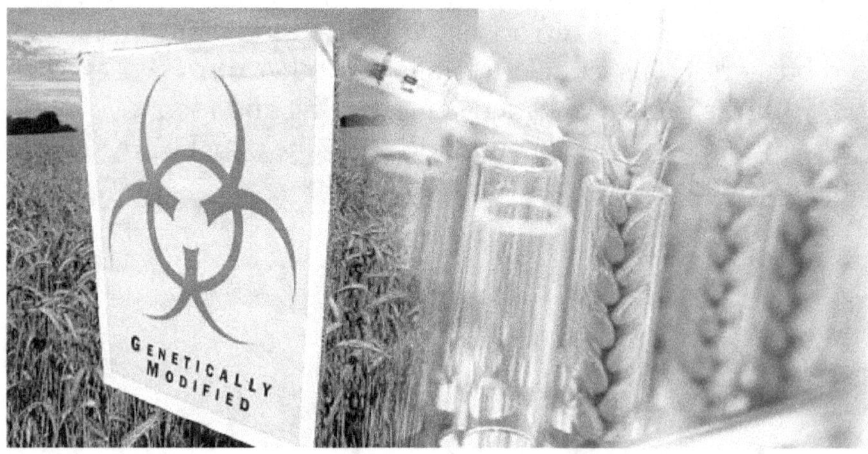

Wheat, the iconic amber wave of grain and a principal staple cereal and flour product in human history and culture, moved onto the endangered list of natural and organic heritage grains at the end of 2023 and early 2024 as the world's first genetically modified wheat (GMO) was produced in Argentina.

Known as HB4 and modified to tolerate drought and fight climate change, the new transgenic variety produced by Bioceres has been approved for import into Brazil, Uruguay, Paraguay, Nigeria, South Africa, Australia, New Zealand, Colombia, and Indonesia. The U.S. FDA concluded two years ago that GMO wheat was safe for consumption, but approval for planting is pending at the U.S. Department of Agriculture.

The release of the Argentine variety rolls back 25 years' of successful efforts by health and environmental organizations around the world to prevent its commercialization. Following its debut, a coalition of small farm, ecology, and indigenous organizations from Latin America, Africa, and Asia requested that the United Nations intervene and halt its use to protect food sovereignty and nutritional security around the world.

The planting and consumption of the new altered wheat, the coalition charged, violates several human rights such as the right to life and livelihoods; health; a balanced and pollution-free environment; access to land and territory; and the right to self-determination of peoples and local communities that survive off the environment and nature, especially in marginal lands that are targeted by the new drought-resistance variety.

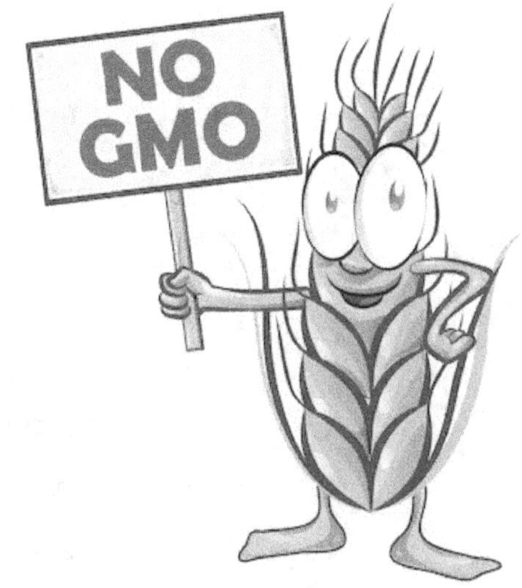

More than a thousand scientists associated with Conicet, the main Argentine research agency, and thirty public universities in Argentina, condemned the approval of the HB4 wheat and warned of the risks to the health of the population.

"This authorization refers to an agribusiness model that has proven to be harmful in environmental and social terms, is the main cause of biodiversity loss, does not solve food problems, and further threatens the health of our people threatening food security and sovereignty," the open letter to the government and company began.

HB4 wheat not only contains inserted sunflower genes to increase tolerance to drought, but also it has been altered to be resistant to the herbicide glufosinate ammonium, a pesticide that has been banned, due to its high toxicity, in many other countries. The EU classified it as toxic to the reproductive system.

Big Ag companies such as Bioceres claim that their products will reduce pesticide use. But the introduction of herbicide-resistant transgenic monocultures has produced herbicide-resistant weeds. To maintain yields, stronger, more toxic chemicals are sprayed on crops rather than less. In Brazil, for example, pesticide use increased 3.4% between 2008 when GMO maize was first cultivated and 2022. Similar hikes have occurred with other engineered crops and could be expected in transgenic wheat.

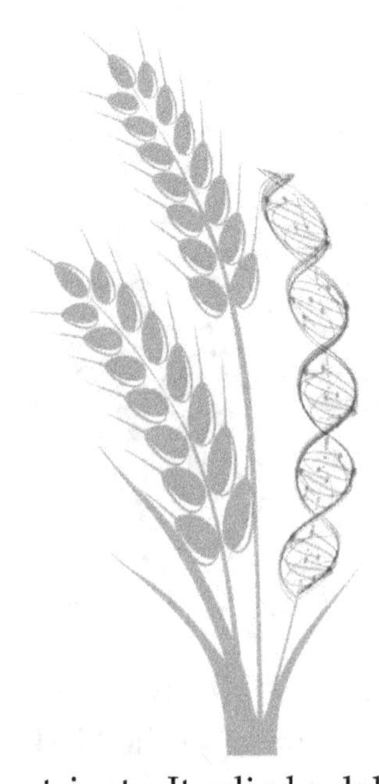

As for the higher yields, Bioceres promised, data from the Argentine Ministry of Agriculture showed that in the 2021/2022 growing season, experimental HB4 yielded 17% less than ordinary wheat fields. Critics charged the country with approving the new altered strain behind closed doors and without publishing any peer reviewed scientific studies.

Argentine regulators did not carry out any experimental tests to determine whether gene modification could lead to an increase in toxic metabolites, anti-nutrients or allergens, or a decrease in important nutrients. It relied solely on the technical-scientific information submitted by Bioceres based, according to government documents, on "the principle of good faith." Nor was there any consultation with local or indigenous communities in "marginal" areas where the drought-resistant strain would be planted.

Bioceres reported that already 25 flour mills were combining GM wheat with conventional wheat for free distribution. Giving away free food and seeds is a tactic biotech companies often use to spread their new wares. Later, they require farmers to purchase new patented GMO seeds each year at premium prices. Farmers that replant company seeds are arrested and subject to heavy fines.

As Vandana Shiva, a leader of the global movement for sustainable agriculture, has documented, GMO crops have bankrupted many small farmers and their families in India, Africa, and other regions of the Global South. It has led to waves of suicides in the face of GMO crop failures, destitution, and starvation.

In Argentina and many countries, there is no GM labeling, so consumers have no way of knowing they are consuming an altered product. As a wheat-exporting country, Argentina ships wheat abroad and poses a threat to other regions. Elizabeth Brava of Accion Ecologica de Ecuador, a neigh-boring country, declared, "Wheat is fundamental to the diet of Ecuadorians, as it is for many other peoples in the world, because it is present from breakfast to dinner. It would be terrible if we started eating wheat that is genetically modified and also has major pesticide residues such as glufosinate ammonium."

"The production model on which HB4 wheat is based is inherently land-grabbing because the costs saved in the use of inputs and labor are justified on large tracts of land," the indigenous coalition further warned. "In addition, aerial spraying prevents the development of other non-GM crops, displaces other ways of working the land, homogenizes landscape with few varieties, and expands monocultures into natural ecosystems."

The representatives from the Southern Cone, as Argentina, Chile, and Uruguay are called, also warned that while wheat is self-pollinating, a small amount can be pollinated by insects or air currents and contaminate conventional or organic varieties. Seed drills, combines, and other farm equipment, storage units, and transportation vehicles could also mix grains and unintentionally contaminate regular crops and the food supply.

Noting that agribusiness is responsible for up to 37% of global carbon dioxide emissions, the non-GMO alliance concluded that the spread of GMO wheat could lead to "a real chemical war being waged against rural communities and nature, deterioration of the health of the population, advance of deforestation, grabbing of public and collective lands, and violence against local communities." The alliance said HB4 was part of the "scorched earth" logic of monocultures to respond to global warming and climate change "akin to trying to put out a fire with gasoline."

Mexico Protects Its Maize Heritage

In 2020, Mexico pledged to phase out GMO corn imports from the United States and prohibit the use of glyphosate, the herbicide that accompanies many altered crops, by 2024. Maize, which first grew in Mexico and is intertwined with its culture, means "source of life."

The Biden Administration is now fighting back and demanding that the country lift its bans and accept genetically engin-

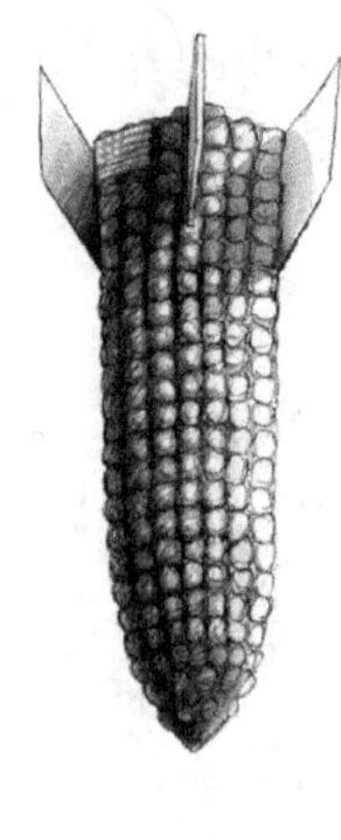

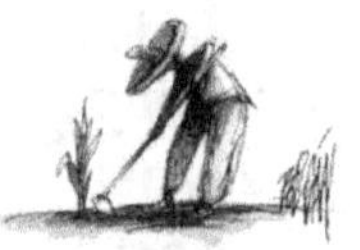

eered corn and glyphosate that has been banned in many parts of the world. Developed by Monsanto and sold under the name Roundup Ready, glyphosate is a probable carcinogen according to the World Health Organization. It is the subject of recent billion-dollar legal judgments in favor of farmers, gardeners, and others who contracted cancer from exposure to spraying it on their fields and gardens.

The NAFTA (North American Free Trade Alliance) in the mid-1990s allowed unrestricted agricultural trade between the U.S., Mexico, and Canada. Following the introduction of GMO corn in the U.S. in the early 2000s, the Commission on Environmental Cooperation warned: "Impacts on the genetic diversity of Mexican maize could have direct repercussions on the diversity of maize and ecosystems in all of North America and the rest of the world. Mexico is one of the centers of origin for maize. To lose a variety of maize in Mexico is to lose it throughout the planet."

In 2023, President Biden issued an executive order making genetic engineering a national priority. "Biotechnology and biomanufacturing are providing transformative solutions to many of the greatest challenges facing U.S. agriculture and food production, including climate change, food and nutritional security, and pests and diseases in agricultural plants and animals," the report that accompanied the White House order stated. More food-grade biomanufacturing facilities, including ones for precision fermentation, stepped up gene sequencing of plants and animals and breeding facilities, and promoting greater consumer acceptance of GMO food products were specified.

In the U.S. today, more than 90% of the corn, soybeans, and cotton are genetically engineered.

Challenging Mexico's ban on GMO corn and herbicide, the U.S. charged that it would result in the loss of millions of dollars of agricultural trade and seriously harm American corn

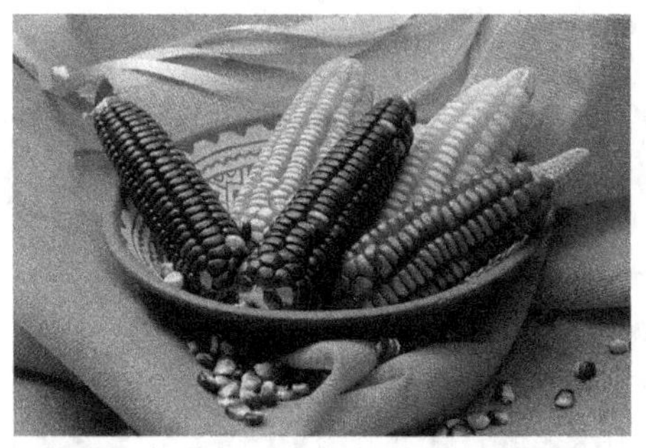

producers. Mexico imported 20 million metric tons of corn from its northern neighbor in 2021-2022. In retaliation, the U.S. threatened to place tariffs on Mexican products exported to the U.S.

In March, Mexican Agriculture Secretary Victor Suarez reiterated that the science shows modified corn and glyphosate are harmful to native maize varieties and human health and that prohibiting them were within Mexico's rights. He challenged the U.S. to produce evidence to the contrary. "But we still haven't seen the science of the United States or the companies We are looking forward to that study with great pleasure."

A largely unrecognized consequence of GMO corn in Mexico has been its impact on the social upheavals, crime, and declining health of the Mexican people. After large amounts of GMO corn entered Mexico in the early 2000s, the price of domestically-grown maize plunged. Unable to make a living, many farmers fled north to the U.S. as legal or illegal immigrants. The rise of drug cartels and waves of kidnappings, disappearances, and other criminal violence in Mexico may also be related to the consumption of GMO corn and its adverse effects on health and consciousness.

Fluttering Close to Extinction

Monarch butterflies, also native to Mexico, are nearing extinction in large part due to GMO crops in North America. During the warmer months, millions of beautiful orange-and-black insects migrate north from California to New England. Milkweed, the only plant on which monarchs lay their eggs and on which monarch cater-pillars feed, has been devastated by Bt and gylphosate, an insecticide and herbicide used on GMO corn, soy, cotton, and other crops.

A survey by the World Wildlife Fund (WWF) this past winter found record-low numbers of Monarchs in their native wintering location in the forests of central Mexico. The insect's

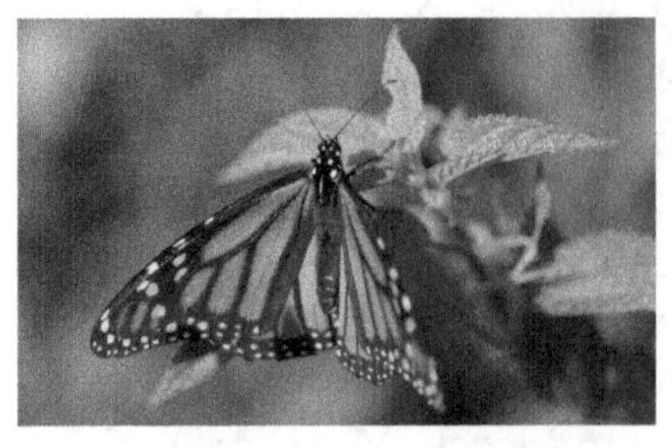

colonies took up just 2.2 acres of forests, 59% less than during the 2022-2023 winter season. "Land-use changes in the United States, combined with the widespread use of herbicides, also contributed to the loss of milkweed and other nectar plants essential to feeding adult monarchs," the WWF reported.

Updates from Europe, Japan, China, and Korea

Early this year the European Parliament approved the use of the New Genomic Techniques (NGT) and exempted 94% of these plants from most GMO safety requirements. NGT utilizes newly developed CRISPR gene-editing technology to genetically combine or alter gene sequences within the *same* species or related species. Conventional GMO crops are produced by combining genes from two or more *different* species. Labeling for seeds would still be required.

The decision undoes 20 years of the "precautionary principles," the GMO-Free Italy Coalition, an alliance of 45 health and environmental groups, stated in opposition to the deregulation. It predicted that Europe would undergo a further concentration of the seed market and a wave of new patents that would negatively impact farmers and consumers.

In Japan, the GABA CRISPR-edites tomato was released in 2023. According to the manufacturer, the tomatoes will lower blood pressure, relieve mental stress, and improve sleep quality. The amount of gamma aminobutyric acid (GABA) in the altered tomatoes was reportedly from 4 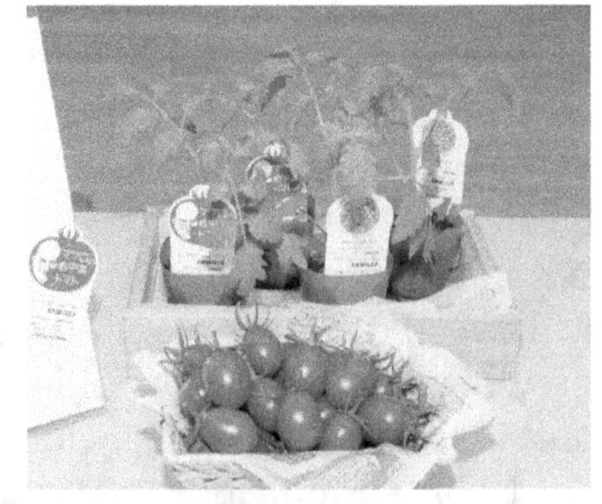 to 6 times higher than in conventionally bred varieties. GABA is the chief inhibitory neurotransmitter in the mammalian central nervous system and reduces neuronal excitability. It is used in drugs to increase relaxation, reduce anxiety, and pevent convulsions. On the downside, GABA can cause increased heart rate, muscle weakness, nausea, headache, and amnesia. Clinical research has found that GABA supplementation did not reduce stress or enhance sleep quality.

In early 2024, China approved additional varieties of GMO soybeans and corn for import and production while expanding their growing area nationwide. The edict includes six new varieties of corn, two of soy, and one of cotton. The agricultural ministry further approved the world's first gene-edited soybeans. Researchers reported that the NGT soybeans boosted yields in temperate regions. The CRISPR soybeans were developed with the help of scientists from Syngenta Biotechnology, one of the world's largest biotech companies. A major producer of Bt corn and soy, the company is based in Basel and was bought by Sinochem, a Chinese state-owned enterprise, in 2017.

In February, the Chinese Academy of Agricultural Science reported using CRISPR on a gene in rice to produce a strain that is more tolerant of salt. No GMO rice is currently commercialized in China or anywhere else in the world.

Golden Rice, the controversial GMO rice developed by the IRRI (International Rice Research Institute) in the Philippines to combat Vitamin-A deficiency in children, was approved for release. But this spring the Supreme Court in the Philippines ruled that all cultivation of Golden Rice (and GMO eggplant) must be stopped until proven safe following the petition from MASIPAG, a network of people's organizations, farmers, and NGOs.

In South Korea, scientists have developed a way to grow beef muscle on rice grains, increasing its protein and fat content. They claim cultured meat offers a solution to famine, can be used as military rations, and has a lower carbon footprint than beef.

CRISPR USA

Following an executive order by President Trump in 2019 to streamline the process, the FDA, USDA, and EPA, which share oversight over genetically engineered foods, determined that gene-edited crops do not have to be regulated because they do not incorporate foreign genes from viruses or bacteria like GMOs.

In the U.S., the first CRISPR gene-edited food was a soybean created in 2019 to yield high oleic

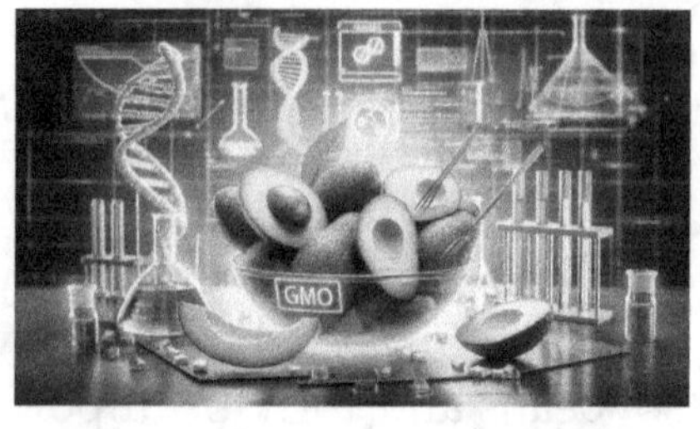

oil and avoid producing trans fats when cooked at high temperatures. Produced by the biotech company Calyxt, the soy oil was slow to be adopted by farmers because of its lower crop yields. Ultimately, it failed, and the company exited the crop commerce business.

Last summer, Pairwise marketed its "Conscious Greens," a mix of purple and green gene-edited mustard greens. It claimed the new blend was designed to taste less bitter and more like lettuce. The Center for Food Safety, an environmental group in Washington, D.C. that opposed its release, expressed concerns that the CRISPR-edited product could lead to chromothripsis in which several hundred genetic changes occur at once and result in diseased plants. A recent study at Cold Spring Harbor Laboratory reported chromothripsis-like effects in experimental gene-edited tomatoes. GreenVenus introduced a non-browning avocado last year using CRISPR.

Brave New NGT World

As the advent of GMO wheat and biotech developments around the globe show, the planet entered a fraught new era of genetically engineered foods this year. Bread, flour, noodles, pasta, cookies, crackers, cakes, and other products made from wheat, the principal food for nearly half the globe, are now imperiled. The war in Ukraine, which has dramatically reduced the amount of wheat available on the world market, has caused hunger in the Middle East, Central Asia, and other regions dependent on imports from Eastern Europe and Russia.

The biotech companies are using the Ukrainian conflict as a pretext for rolling out their new untested and patented wares in the same way they invoke climate change and global warming as excuses to introduce new CRISPR gene-edited foods. A flood

---

of new NGT foods is in the pipeline. Unless resisted by diet- and health-conscious scientists, physicians, parents, children, and other concerned citizens, the natural food supply may reach the point of no return.

Reengineering the bounty of nature that has sustained countless generations from the dawn of our species is not the answer. It will only compound the crises humanity faces. Regenerative natural and organic agriculture continues to offer a safe, viable path to a world of enduring health, peace, and diversity.

*

Observing Nature: The Best Evidence Ever Against GMOs

On a journey through the Corn Belt in the Midwest, a farm journalist reported that cattle wouldn't touch modified corn stubble, hogs wouldn't eat their ration of GMO crops, and raccoons romped by the dozen through the organic corn but left the Bt fields untouched.

One farmer described observing a herd of 40 deer "mowing down his tofu beans while across the road there isn't one doe eating on the Roundup Readies."

"Even the mice will move down the line if given an alternative to these 'crops.' What is it that they know instinctively that most of us ignore?"

— "When the Corn Hits the Fan," *ACRES USA*, Sept. 18, 1999.

Resources

Planetary Health/Amberwaves
Planetary Health is a nonprofit educational organization devoted to macrobiotic education and creating personal and planetary health and peace. Founded in 2000 in the Berkshires by Alex Jack and Edward Esko, it sponsors the Amberwaves grassroots network that has led campaigns against GMO rice, wheat, and other foods, publishes books and a newsletter, engages in medical research, and produces the forthcoming film *The Spirit of Rice*. It also holds online conferences, courses, and dietary and health consultations.
www.planetaryhealth.com

GMWatch
GMWatch provides the latest news and comment on GMO and CRISPR-edited foods and crops and their associated pesticides. Founded in 1998, it is based in the U.K. and covers events worldwide.
www.gmowatch.org

GMO-Free U.S.A. and Toxin-Free U.S.A.
GMO/Toxin Free USA's mission is to harness independent science and agroecological concepts to advocate for clean and healthy food and ecological systems. A Connecticut-based organization founded in 2012 that organizes national boycotts of food companies that use GMO ingredients and pressures them to remove them. Its initiatives include Boycott Kellogg's GMOs campaign and another aimed at Whole Foods for selling GMO sweet corn. In 2020, it expanded its focus beyond GMOs to "clean food and the environment" and established Toxin Free USA.
www.toxinfreeusa.org

GRAIN
GRAIN is a small international non-profit organization based in Barcelona, Spain that works to support small farmers and social movements in their struggles for community-controlled and biodiversity-based food systems, especially in Africa, Asia, and Latin America. It prepares comprehensive reports on organic and sustainable agriculture, the threats of agribusiness, climate change, and indigenous practices.
www.grain.org

Green America
Green America harnesses economic power—the strength of consumers, investors, businesses, and the marketplace—to create a socially just and environmentally sustainable society. Formerly known as Coop America, the

organization organizes a variety of campaigns, including the Stop GMO
Wheat campaign.
www.greenamerica.org

Navdana

Vandana Shiva's organization in India devoted to arcoecology, organic
farming, seedbanks, and campaigns against GMOs.
www.navdana.org

Non-GMO Project

The Non-GMO Project is a nonprofit organization committed to building
and preserving the non-GMO food supply. As a third-party, it verifies and
labels non-GMO products and makes its database publicly available for
consumers. It was founded by two natural food stores in 2007 and has
verified more than 50,000 products.
www.nongmoproject.org

Organic Consumers Association

OCA educates and advocates on behalf of organic consumers,
engages consumers in marketplace pressure campaigns, and works to
advance sound food and farming policy through grassroots lobbying. It
addresses crucial issues around food safety, industrial agriculture, genetic
engineering, children's health, corporate accountability, Fair Trade,
environmental sustainability, including pesticide use, and other food- and
agriculture-related topics.
www.organicconsumers.org

Organic & Non-GMO Report

Ken Roseboro's publications and web site are devoted to organic food and
regenerative farming. He publishes the *Organic & Non-GMO Sourcebook*, a
buyer's guide to suppliers of non-GMO and organic seed, crops, ingredients,
and food products and a bimonthly *Organic & Non-GMO Report*.
www.non-gmoreport.com

Genetic Literacy Project

A nonprofit that publishes a database of GMO and CRISPR gene-edited
foods by country. Includes hundreds of listings, plus regulations, and articles
on biotechnology. It is pro-GMO, anti-organic, and pro-pharma, but its
database is comprehensive and up-to-date.
www.geneticliteraryproject.org

Amberwaves Press

   Selected books from Amberwaves on GMOs, organic farming, and related topics.

Biowisdom by Alex Jack, $12.95. "Biowisdom" is the intuitive understanding of what is necessary, right, and appropriate for sustaining life on the planet. Antonym: biotechnology, bioterrorism, bioreactor. Includes natural approaches to protect against radiation, develop your intuition, and awaken you to approaching danger and strengthen your spirit. Includes Dennis Kucinich's proposal for a Department of Peace.

Growing Rice in Your Backyard by Wayne Weber, $10.00. Dry land rice will grow almost anywhere without the need for special irrigation. This book shows how to get started.

Healing with Rice by Alex and Gale Jack, $14.95. Includes over 100 special dishes, medicinal drinks, and compresses to maintain optimal health, a calm, peaceful mind, and prevent and relieve illness.

Humanity at a Wireless Crossroads by Cynthia Vann, $12.95. Everything you need to know about cell phones; electric, microwave, and induction cooking; hearing aids; electric vehicles, smart meters, and the impact of EMFs (electro-magnetic fields) on your health and well-being. *"I'm very impressed with the easy-to-understand technical presentations in these articles. Read this book, it will open your mind to new ideas about things you thought you knew."* —James Sharp, former Naval Quality Analyst in the Quality Evaluation Laboratory, Seal Beach, CA

Imagine a World Without Monarch Butterflies: Awakening to the Hazards of Genetically Altered Foods by Alex Jack, $10.95. Summary of the major health and environmental dangers of GMO foods. *"A powerful compendium of well-researched information which is essential reading for anyone who wants to understand the awesome challenge which GE foods present to all of humanity." – Congressman Dennis J. Kucinich, from the foreword*

Living on Earth by Abraham Oort, $35.00. In this memoir, a meteorologist at the Geophysical Fluid Dynamics Laboratory in Princeton, NJ, describes his life researching the Earth's climate and its unexpected, rapid recent changes. He later taught shiatsu at the Kushi Institute, studied Buddhist mindfulness and meditation with Thich Nhat Hanh, and continued his search for personal freedom and a solution to the global climate crisis.

Out of Thin Air by Alex Jack, $12.95. A hilarious courtroom drama set in the globally warmed 21st century in which an advertising executive is brought to trial for refusing to pay the $15,000 environmental tax for eating a hamburger. *"With a wide array of bioregional witnesses and a jury of endangered species, the modern diet is put on trial. Funny and affecting." – Vegetarian Times*

———

The Rice Revolution by Four Organic Farmers, $00.00. Several farmers in the Northeast independently started growing rice, sharing seeds, and promoting local rice cultivation. Christian Elwell, founder of South River Miso, started growing rice nearly thirty years ago in western Massachusetts. Takeshi Akaogi, a farmer from Japan, who studied with Masanobu Fukuoka, author of The One-Straw Revolution, started growing rice in Vermont. Eric Andrus, a wheat farmer in the Champlain Valley of Vermont, began to grow organic rice at Boundbrook Farm. In Maine, Ben Rooney started growing rice at Wild Folk Farm.

Saving Organic Rice edited by Alex Jack and Edward Esko, $10.95. Articles on the threat of genetically engineered rice to organic rice, wheat, and other crops by Dr. Vandana Shiva, Dr. Mae-Wan Ho, Paul Hawken, and other scientists and environmentalists. *"This one slender volume gathers the insights of some of the world's leading proponents of sustainable agriculture and ecological balance." – Nina Molliver*

Vanishing Rice Fields by Alex Jack, $10.95. Protecting the world's #1 crop from global warming and climate change.

Books are available from Amberwaves, Box 487, Becket MA 01223. Please add $5.95 postage in the U.S. Foreign airmail will be billed at cost.

Notes

1. Press Release: The American Academy of Environmental Medicine, May 19, 2009. www.aaemonline.org/gmopressrelease.html.

2. P. Hepsomali, (2020). "Effects of Oral Gamma-Aminobutyric Acid (GABA) Administration on Stress and Sleep in Humans," Front Neurosci. 14: 923

3. "CRISPR causes serious DNA damage with high frequency – but it's often overlooked," www.gmwatch.org, August 9, 2023.

4. Ibid.

5. "CRISPR gene editing causes whole chromosome loss," www.gmwatch.org, November 19, 2021.

6. Ibid.

7. See Alex Jack, *Imagine a World without Monarch Butterflies* for a summary of scores of medical studies documenting these 50 concerns.

8. Robert Hatherill, Editorial, *Chicago Tribune*, June 15, 1999; "Study Urged of Pesticide, Youth Violence Link," Environmental News Network, August 9, 1999.

9. Scott C. Yates, "GMO Fight Comes to Supplements Aisle," *Natural Foods Merchandiser*, October 2000.

10. Don Campbell, *The Mozart Effect*, Avon Books, New York, 1997.

11. Nina Moliver quoted in Alex Jack, *Imagine a World Without Monarch Butterflies*, 2000, pp. 48-49.

12. Stephen R. Padgette et al., "The Composition of Glyphosate Tolerant Soybean Seeds Is Equivalent to That of Conventional Soybeans," *Journal of Nutrition* 126:4, 1996.

13. Naaz Modan and Kara Arundel, "School shootings reach unprecedented high in 2022," www.k12dive.com, Dec. 21, 2022.

14. There's been an on-campus shooting "pretty much every single school day" this fall, the founder of the K-12 School Shooting Database said.

15. M. M. Lane et al, "Ultra-processed food exposure and adverse health outcomes: umbrella review of epidemiological meta-analyses," *BMJ* 2024.

About the Author

Alex Jack is an author, teacher, and macrobiotic dietary counselor. He has served as a civil rights worker in Mississippi, Vietnam War correspondent, editor-in-chief of *East West Journal*, executive director of Kushi Institute, and president of Planetary Health, Inc.

He serves on the guest faculty of Rosas Dance Company in Brussels, the Escola Macrobiótica in Portugal, and the Ohsawa Center in Tokyo. He has also presented at the Zen Temple in Beijing, the Cardiology Institute of St. Petersburg, and Shake-speare's New Globe Theatre in London.

His books include *The Cancer Prevention Diet, One Peaceful World,* and *The Gospel of Peace: Jesus's Teachings of Eternal Truth* with Michio Kushi; *The Mozart Effect: Tapping the Power of Music to Heal the Body, Strengthen the Mind, and Unlock the Creative Spirit* with Don Campbell; editions and commentaries on *Hamlet* and *As You Like It* by Christopher Marlowe and William Shake-speare.

Alex lives in Slovakia with his wife, Danka. He has a daughter who has an organic farm in Russia and five grandchildren.

Contact: shenwa26@yahoo.com • www.planetaryhealth.com